THE ULTIMATE GASTRITIS GUIDE & COOKBOOK

120 Delicious Gluten-Free and Dairy-Free Recipes for the Treatment, Prevention and Cure of Gastritis

PAUL HIGGINS

Copyright © 2017 by Paul Higgins. All rights reserved.

No part of *The Ultimate Gastritis Guide & Cookbook* shall be reproduced, resold, reprinted or stored in a retrieval system, or transmitted in any form or by any means, including electronic, mechanical, photocopying, recording or otherwise, without the written permission of the author. This work is copyrighted and any unauthorized use of its contents is strictly prohibited.

DISCLAIMER OF LIABILITY

No liability whatsoever is assumed regarding the use of the information contained in this book. Despite all the precautions taken in the elaboration of this book, neither the author nor its partners/affiliates assume any liability for errors, inaccuracies or omissions. Nor shall any liability be assumed for damages resulting from the use of the information found in this book. The information in it is for informative use only.

Any slight to individuals or organizations is involuntary, unintentional. The information provided is on a "as it is" basis, and if you need legal or medical advice, or connected in any way to this publication, you should seek the services of a fully qualified professional. This book is not designed in any way to be used as a source of medical advice. Anyone who reads this guide must agree with the statements made in this legal notice.

ISBN-13: 978-1979024136 | eBook ISBN: B076JHWC77

Printed in the United States of America

First Edition: October 2017

Second Edition: June 2020

TABLE OF CONTENTS

Introduction 9

PART 1: GETTING STARTED

Chapter 1: WHAT IS GASTRITIS?............................. 15
Chapter 2: UNDERSTANDING THE STOMACH 21
Chapter 3: WHAT IS RUINING YOUR STOMACH?..... 27

PART 2: TREATING AND RELIEVING GASTRITIS

Chapter 4: THE GASTRITIS DIET................................ 33
Chapter 5: SUPPLEMENTS AND REMEDIES 43

PART 3: THE RECIPES

Chapter 6: BREAKFAST RECIPES............................. 55
    Simple Oatmeal 56
    Blueberry Banana Smoothie Bowl.......................... 57
    Spinach Mushroom Scrambled Eggs 58
    Pumpkin Spinach Smoothie 59
    Buckwheat Waffles... 60
    Blueberry Almond Smoothie 62
    Chia Rice Pudding 63
    Banana Oat Pancakes... 64
    Stewed Apples & Blueberries 65
    French Toast 66

Rice Porridge 67
Coconut Flour Pumpkin Pancakes 68
Apple Pie Quinoa Porridge 70
Rice Banana Waffles... 71
Banana Chia Seed Custard...................................... 72
Sweet Potato Pancakes 74
Coconut Bread... 76
Banana Bread 77
Buckwheat & Quinoa Porridge 78
Blueberry Muffins... 80
Blueberry Chia Pudding 82
Coconut Quinoa Porridge 83
Banana Crumble.. 84
Turkey Breakfast Sausage....................................... 85
Coconut Almond Cereal 86

Chapter 7: POULTRY & SEAFOOD RECIPES 89

Chicken & Veggie Stir-Fry...................................... 90
Grilled Salmon with Yogurt Sauce 92
Crispy Baked Cod 93
Herbed Grilled Tuna Steaks.................................... 94
Baked Fish with Carrots 95
Crab Cakes 96
Grilled Chicken with Kale....................................... 98
Vegetable Turkey Stew 100
Baked Fish with Thyme Crusted...........................101
Grilled Prawn Skewers 102
Tilapia with Sautéed Kale 103
Broiled Shrimp...104
Maple-Glazed Scallops 105

Grilled Chicken with Spinach 106

Turkey with Kale 107

Chicken & Red Lentils Stew 108

Veggie Loaded Meatloaf 109

Baked Salmon with Avocado.................................110

Baked Turkey Meatballs 111

Creamy Chicken & Broccoli Casserole 112

Zucchini Shrimp Scampi 114

Coconut Chicken with Spinach 115

Baked Portobello & Salmon 116

Shrimp Avocado Omelette 118

Almond Crusted Tilapia 120

Chicken Zucchini Meatballs 121

Coconut Fish Sticks...122

Turkey Quinoa Meatloaf..123

Zucchini Wrapped Fish 124

Turkey Broccoli & Rice Casserole..........................126

Chapter 8: SALAD & SOUP RECIPES........................ 129

Apple Walnut Kale Salad 130

Carrot Waldorf Salad...131

Avocado Mango Broccoli Salad 132

Fresh Fruit Salad 133

Moroccan Carrot & Spinach Salad.........................134

Apple & Carrot Salad...135

Quinoa & Kale Salad 136

Ginger-Sesame Veggie Salad 138

Avocado Egg Salad 139

Herbed Summer Squash Salad..............................140

Kale & Zucchini Soup 141

Creamy Broccoli Soup 142

Pumpkin & Sweet Potato Soup 143

Chicken & Kale Soup 144

Lentil Spinach Soup 145

Chickpeas & Celery Soup..146

Miso Soup 147

Roasted Winter Squash Soup 148

Creamy Carrot Soup 150

Creamy Shrimp & Rice Soup..................................151

Chapter 9: SIDE DISH & VEGAN RECIPES 153

Butternut Squash and Kale 154

Squashes & Chickpeas..155

Roasted Broccoli Chickpea Quinoa 156

Roasted Tofu & Vegetables.....................................158

Chickpea Kale & Quinoa Stew 160

Sautéed Potatoes 162

Red Lentils & Veggie Stew 163

Tofu with Red Lentils 164

White & Wild Rice Pilaf...165

Carrot Patties 166

Roasted Carrots & Fennel 167

Tofu Quinoa Stir Fry 168

Tofu Vegetable Scramble 170

Mushrooms & Quinoa Pilaf 172

Rice and Lentil Pilaf..174

Veggie Patties 176

Roasted Sweet Potatoes 177

Crunchy Cauliflower Casserole 178

Zucchini and Potato Bake 179

Kale and Coconut Stir Fry.................................180
Spinach Mashed Potatoes...............................182

Chapter 10: SNACKS & SWEETS RECIPES 183

Cauliflower Salmon Bites 184
Carrot Cake Balls 185
Sweet Potato Biscuits 186
Baked Zucchini Fries 188
Avocado Wedges 189
Pretzel Sticks 190
Avocado Carob Pudding 192
Baked Potato Chips 193
Banana Oat Bars 194
Banana "Nice" Cream 195
Herbed Crackers...196
Coconut Almond Butter Bars 198
Buckwheat Muffins 200
Coconut Crackers & Sticks 202
Coconut Clouds 204

Chapter 11: ANTI-INFLAMMATORY SMOOTHIES.....205

Banana Spinach Smoothie..............................206
Papaya Mango Smoothie 207
Carrot Banana Smoothie 208
Berry Beet Smoothie 210
Papaya Green Smoothie 211
Blueberry Spinach Smoothie 212
Avocado Berry Smoothie 213
Apple Green Smoothie 214
Carrot Mango Smoothie 215
Ginger Berry Smoothie 216

Chapter 12: EXTRA RECIPES 217
    Homemade Non-Dairy Milk 218
    Homemade Coconut Yogurt 220
    Homemade Almond Milk Yogurt 223
    Homemade Chicken Broth 226
    Homemade Vegetable Broth 228

THE ACTION PLAN 229
ABOUT THE AUTHOR 238

INTRODUCTION

One of the worst things you can experience when you are suffering with gastritis is the burning that goes from your stomach to your esophagus. You feel very uncomfortable and as though you don't want to do anything more than take or drink something for immediate relief.

Maybe you are wondering whether this is how the rest of your life is going to be. And I know, from experience, that when you live with annoying symptoms, life is nothing less than abject misery. And it is also very unpleasant to think that this is how your life is going to be forever.

I know how you are feeling right now. You are maybe tired of having to avoid your favorite foods or drinks; tired of avoiding to go out with friends or family for fear of eating or drinking something what would cause you a gastritis attack; or tired of having to deal with those annoying symptoms every single day. But don't worry, I feel your pain and I can tell you that you are definitely not alone.

Gastritis is a common digestive disorder that affects millions of people around the world, and thousands of new cases are reported worldwide every year.

However, many people are not well-informed about what to eat, which foods can worsen or improve their gastritis, and what lifestyle changes they must make in order to heal their stomachs.

And as you know, learning about how to eat for a particular health problem can take a lot of time if you research it on your own. You also might have trouble differentiating between good and bad information. Sometimes even having the right information is not enough because you face other problems, like cravings that make it difficult to comply with a strict diet.

For that reason, this book has been created so that you do not have to spend months researching about this condition and can stick to the gastritis diet as long as you needed to allow your stomach to heal.

In *The Ultimate Gastritis Guide & Cookbook* you will discover more than 120 gastritis-friendly recipes and all you need to know about this condition—including dietary and lifestyle choices to help you heal your stomach. The recipes you will find are delicious and make excellent substitutes for some of those cravings or foods you love. This means you will be less likely to yield to those cravings. It also includes recipes for snacks and desserts you can enjoy without having to worry about gastritis.

This is more than a simple recipe book; it is your complete guide to living a healthier and happier life by safely reducing and relieving your symptoms and stomach problems.

HOW TO USE THIS BOOK

I have separated this book into three parts and several chapters. I suggest that you read all chapters once and then use the information as a reference to which you can refer back in the future. Here's what you'll find in this book:

The first (page 15) and second chapter (page 21) give you a detailed introduction to gastritis and how the gastrointestinal system works.

In the third chapter (page 27) you will also learn about some foods and eating habits that can worse your gastritis and trigger symptoms. It is important to know the problem very well —as well as to know what is causing it— as having this knowledge can be very useful when you are creating a therapeutic strategy for treating and healing gastritis.

The fourth chapter (page 33) introduces you to the gastritis diet, which includes a list of foods you should avoid and include in your diet. You'll also find a list of recommendations and tips.

In the fifth chapter (page 43) you will find a list of supplements and natural remedies for gastritis. Researches have proven that these supplements and natural remedies have regenerative, soothing, protective and anti-inflammatory effects on the stomach lining and that are effective to treat digestive problems such as gastric ulcers and gastritis.

The sixth chapter (page 55) and beyond contains the recipes for gastritis ranging from breakfast to lunches, dinner, snacks, and desserts. You will also find some homemade recipes to make your own non-dairy milks or yogurts, and broths that you can use in recipes calling for it. All the recipes have been specifically created taking into account irritating ingredients that can irritate the stomach lining. You can use the recipes as they are, or customize them to your liking.

In the end of this book (page 229) you will find an action plan and one-week meal plan with its respective shopping list and tips for meal prep. You can customize the meal plan in your own way or use it as inspiration to create your own weekly meal plan.

My intention in writing this book is to give basic, easy-to-understand information to anyone newly diagnosed with gastritis or who has been suffering for years. I really hope you find something helpful in these pages, whether it's a new recipe, new information, or a new point of view.

PART ONE

GETTING STARTED

CHAPTER 1

WHAT IS GASTRITIS?

Gastritis is a common disease of the digestive system. It occurs when the stomach lining becomes inflamed after it's been damaged. It's usually mild and improves quickly if treated. But if not, it can last for years.

The diagnosis of gastritis is histological. This means it is necessary to introduce an endoscope through the patient's esophagus so as to see the stomach's condition and to obtain samples of the stomach lining through a biopsy. Therefore, the diagnosis of gastritis is not only clinical; it is necessary to perform invasive tests (endoscopy and biopsy) to confirm its existence.

Types of Gastritis

There are different types of gastritis but, in general, gastritis can be classified as being either acute or chronic. The difference between these two is determined by the condition and causes of inflammation. The most common aspect of each type of gastritis is irritation and consequent damage of the stomach lining.

Acute Gastritis

This is one of the most common types of gastritis and is characterized by superficial or deep inflammation of the stomach lining. When we talk about acute gastritis, we are referring to an inflammation of the stomach that occurs suddenly and lasts for a short period of time.

The symptoms of gastritis can be very severe and cause a lot of pain, but they may be short-lived. In some cases, there may be no symptoms (asymptomatic).

Chronic Gastritis

This is the second most common type of gastritis and is characterized by long-term inflammation of the stomach. The term "chronic" refers to the fact that it occurs gradually (throughout months or years), causing degradation of the stomach lining.

Some people do not experience discomfort or symptoms during the first few months. Then, suddenly, symptoms appear which can be moderate or severe. When this type of gastritis is not treated, it can lead to other, more serious complications, such as gastric ulcers, stomach bleeding and even cancer.

Atrophic Gastritis

This is a type of gastritis that falls into the category of chronic because it develops over a prolonged period of time and is characterized by the gradual loss of gastric gland cells, which are replaced by other, similar cells which are found in the interior of the intestine (epithelium). When this happens, the stomach lining becomes thinner and more sensitive to external agents, such as bacteria, drugs and irritating foods.

Other Types of Gastritis

There are other types of gastritis, like erosive gastritis, which is characterized by the appearance in the stomach lining of small lesions that can become stomach ulcers. Also, hemorrhagic gastritis can be said to be the next step of erosive gastritis, as ulcers in the stomach can lead to hemorrhages and bleeding in the stomach.

Autoimmune gastritis is due to the stomach lining being attacked by the immune system itself. Other, less common causes are phlegmonous gastritis, which is a fairly rare but potentially dangerous form of acute gastritis characterized by suppurative inflammation and damage to the stomach lining. People with weakened immune systems are more likely to suffer from this type of gastritis.

Symptoms of Gastritis

The symptoms of gastritis may vary from person to person and in terms of the underlying cause. Although some people may have no symptoms, others may experience such symptoms as:

- Stomach or abdominal pain
- Loss of appetite
- Vomiting
- Diarrhea and indigestion
- Nausea
- Dark stools
- Fatigue
- Belching and gas
- Difficulty breathing
- Swelling or feeling of fullness
- Heartburn
- Chest pain

As mentioned above, gastritis affects everyone differently, with symptoms ranging from mild to severe. Some people do not experience any symptoms at all.

Causes of Gastritis

There are many possible causes of gastritis, and these can vary based on the type of gastritis (acute or chronic). Therefore, it is always advisable to consult with a doctor to try to identify the cause of the problem. From the beginning, you should work on finding the cause of gastritis, as the proper treatment will depend on what is causing it.

The various causes are related to the type of gastritis (acute or chronic); for this reason, the causes of acute and chronic gastritis have been separated, and classified as being among the most and less common.

The main causes of acute gastritis are:

- Certain medications such as acetylsalicylic acid (aspirin), ibuprofen, non-steroidal anti-inflammatory drugs (NSAIDs) and corticosteroids.
- Excessive consumption of alcohol and caffeine.
- Infection of the stomach by the bacteria *Helicobacter pylori*.
- Stress (decreases gastric secretions).

Other, less common causes are:

- Viral infections caused by viruses such as *cytomegalovirus* herpes simplex virus (occurs more often in people with weak immune systems).
- Ingestion of corrosive or caustic substances (such as lye, acids or poisons).
- Recreational drugs (e.g., cocaine).

In many cases of gastritis, especially in the chronic type, the patient does not completely know the cause of his or her problem because the patient may have been suffering from it for years without realizing it. However, many of the causes that lead to the onset of chronic gastritis are the same as those that cause the onset of acute gastritis.

The most common causes of chronic gastritis are:

- Hypochlorhydria (low stomach acid).
- Excessive consumption of alcohol.
- *Helicobacter pylori* infection if not treated correctly or if it becomes resistant to antibiotics.

- The consumption of medications such as acetylsalicylic acid (aspirin), ibuprofen, non-steroidal anti-inflammatory drugs (NSAIDs) or corticosteroids.

Other, less common causes are:

- Bile or duodenogastric reflux (including pancreatic juices)
- Autoimmune disorders, which can cause the immune system to attack the stomach cells.
- Digestive disorders such as Crohn's disease, which inflames the digestive tract.
- Pernicious anemia produces chronic atrophic gastritis (autoimmune or type A) in the body and fundus of the stomach.

The reason why some of the factors that cause acute gastritis can cause chronic gastritis too is because once the stomach lining weakens, other substances, such as stomach acid and pepsin, can continue irritating the stomach every time food is ingested.

CHAPTER 2

UNDERSTANDING THE STOMACH

Now that you know what gastritis is, what symptoms it causes, what types of gastritis exist and its causes, let's take a look at how the stomach and the digestive system work.

The stomach is a muscular, elastic, hollow organ of the digestive tract located between the esophagus and duodenum. It also has two sphincters: the lower esophageal sphincter that separates the stomach from the esophagus and the pyloric sphincter that separates the stomach from the duodenum.

The stomach's interior is covered by stomach lining and glands containing various cells that secrete the different substances composing gastric juices (e.g., hydrochloric acid, pepsin, intrinsic factor and gastric mucus). Some of this organ's functions include mixing the food bolus with the gastric juices and temporarily storing broken-down food.

How is Digestion Carried Out?

As soon as you put a piece of food in your mouth, digestion and the secretion of gastric juices begin. Teeth crush food into smaller pieces, which facilitates digestion in the stomach. As the food is chewed, it mixes with the saliva that comes out of the salivary glands. This lubricates the food and facilitates its descent through the esophagus.

> *"Saliva contains different enzymes, but the most abundant is alpha-amylase. This enzyme helps to break down starch into small sugar molecules as they pass through the stomach. Alpha-amylase is deactivated upon contact with stomach acid, allowing other substances to carry out digestion of food."*

The tongue helps move the chewed food towards the bottom of the mouth, where it reaches the pharynx and is propelled towards the stomach. While the food is in the mouth, you can swallow and move your tongue to push the food toward the throat. At this point, digestion is still voluntary; however, once the food passes through the larynx, the involuntary process begins and control over digestion is lost.

A wave-like movement known as peristalsis pushes food through the esophagus. However, before it passes into the stomach, the food travels through the lower esophageal sphincter, which normally opens to admit food or liquids and prevent them from going up to the esophagus.

Digestion in the Stomach

The stomach stores the food after it goes through the esophagus. As you know, one of its functions is to temporarily store food. During that time, gastric contractions continuously push the food. This movement mixes the food with various enzymes and digestive juices – for example, the stomach acid that denatures the proteins and the pepsin to break them down into peptides and amino acids. This process results in a mixture called chyme.

> "Chyme is a semi-fluid consisting of partially digested food, gastric juices and digestive enzymes. This semi-fluid passes from the stomach to the duodenum so that the nutrients it contains are absorbed."

Stomach acid also destroys the various microorganisms we consume with food. This acid is so strong (pH below 1) that it can eliminate any bacteria, parasite or fungus that tries to enter our organisms through the food.

At the end of the stomach we find the pyloric valve, which helps control the gastric emptying towards the duodenum. This sphincter prevents food from returning to the stomach. The time it takes for ingested food to travel from the stomach to the small intestine depends on several factors related to the nature (liquid or solid) or composition (fats or carbohydrates) of the food, as well as the body signals that some hormones emit and the amount of food itself.

When the stomach is empty, water takes 10 to 20 minutes to pass into the duodenum, while larger food particles usually do not pass into the duodenum until they are sufficiently crumbly. The particles must be smaller than 2 millimeters, although generally they are less than 0.25 millimeters before this happens. Solid foods remain in the stomach between one and six hours.

Digestion in the Small Intestine

Once the chyme (which is actually acidic) reaches the duodenum, it is mixed with bile and pancreatic juices to neutralize its acidity and emulsify the fat particles. Pancreatic enzymes are also mixed with the acid chyme to convert small fat particles into lipids, protein into amino acids and carbohydrates into glucose.

The small intestine is the longest part of the digestive system (measuring almost six meters) and is responsible for 90% of food digestion and nutrient absorption. It is divided into three parts: duodenum, jejunum, and ileum.

The duodenum is the initial and shortest section. Its main objective is to further break down partially digested foods with the enzymes the pancreas releases. The duodenum absorbs most of the iron you need.

The jejunum is replete with cells that absorb protein and carbohydrate molecules. Glucose, lipids and amino acids are absorbed through the jejunum's wall into the bloodstream, as well as vitamins, minerals, electrolytes, water and bile salts. The spaces between the jejunum cells are relatively widely separated, making it the most porous section of the small intestine.

The last part of the small intestine is the ileum. This is less porous and absorbent. However, a small proportion of nutrients are absorbed there, including vitamin B12, bile salts and amino acids. At the end of the small intestine is the ileocecal valve that connects the ileum to the large intestine. This valve —like those mentioned previously— prevents food waste from returning to the ileum. Finally, the large intestine carries these "non-digestible" remains into the colon for excretion.

CHAPTER 3

WHAT IS RUINING YOUR STOMACH?

It is interesting to know about the factors that can worsen your gastritis and that might be holding your stomach back from healing. Having such knowledge can be very useful when creating a therapeutic treatment plan to heal your stomach.

Your Eating Habits

Bad eating habits affect not only your health, but also your physical appearance and mood. Consuming foods rich in refined carbohydrates, sugars or saturated fats increases the chances that you will suffer from health conditions that can be difficult to treat or control.

- **Not chewing food:** When you do not chew food properly, it falls like a "stone" to the stomach. This causes the stomach to work harder and food to stay there longer.
- **Not eating at the right time or skipping meals:** Have a specific hour during which you eat your meals and do not

skip meals, as this allows gastric juices to irritate your stomach lining due to a lack of food in your stomach.

- **Eating processed carbohydrates and high-fat foods:** Excessive consumption of foods rich in sugars and processed carbohydrates greatly elevates your stomach pH. Therefore, your stomach must expend a lot of energy to acidify the stomach contents again. Meanwhile, fatty foods slow the gastric emptying and increase inflammation in the stomach. The longer the digestion, the more the stomach lining is exposed to mechanical irritation and stomach acid.

- **Drinking caffeinated beverages:** Excessive consumption of beverages containing caffeine irritates the stomach lining and contributes to the onset of gastritis. Coffee, energy drinks and carbonated drinks are among such beverages.

- **Drinking water while eating:** If you drink water or any liquid while eating, you are diluting your gastric juices, so your stomach must create more acid and enzymes to digest food. If this happens regularly, the cells that secrete gastric juices can get tired and run out of nutrients. In the long run this can cause digestive problems.

Your Lifestyle

Today, many people (unconsciously) follow certain habits that lead to the slow deterioration of their health. In the long run, this can result in diseases or serious health conditions.

- **A stressful life:** Stress can negatively affect digestion by decreasing the body's parasympathetic activity and increasing its sympathetic activity (activated by the stress hormones cortisol and adrenaline). This causes a decrease in gastric secretions. A deficiency of gastric juices can result in the low production of gastric mucus, leaving the stomach lining unprotected and prone to external factors or to its own secretions, causing inflammation and irritation.
- **Smoking:** The nicotine in cigarettes increases the production of stomach acid, which in turn irritates and causes inflammation of the stomach lining.
- **Alcohol:** Alcohol consumption causes the stomach lining to become inflamed. This inflammation is likely to occur if alcohol is regularly consumed. If the consumption is excessive, the stomach does not have the opportunity to recover from the irritation. This can lead to the onset of gastritis.

Your Own Stomach Acid and Pepsin

As you have just read, both the hydrochloric acid your stomach produces and the proteolytic enzyme called pepsin are the main products of gastric secretion capable of inducing mucosal injury. You may be wondering how this is possible. Let me explain.

Stomach acid is a highly corrosive substance (pH below 1) secreted by the stomach's parietal cells. The main role of stomach acid is to break down food, convert pepsinogen into its active form (pepsin) and protect the body from diseases by killing pathogens commonly found in food. Stomach acid accounts for 3-5% of total gastric juices.

On the other hand, pepsin is a proteolytic enzyme secreted by the gastric chief cells in the stomach. This enzyme breaks down proteins into smaller pieces (peptides and amino acids), without completely degrading it—a function performed by other enzymes in the intestine.

The problem with these two substances is that once gastritis occurs, neither allow your stomach to fully recover because every time you eat something (mainly foods rich in proteins), these substances are released and continue irritating the stomach lining.

PART TWO

TREATING AND RELIEVING GASTRITIS

CHAPTER 4

GETTING STARTED WITH THE GASTRITIS DIET

The first step in decreasing inflammation of the stomach is to change your diet. Therefore, the diet for gastritis should consist of foods that are anti-inflammatory, bland, and low-acid. Foods that may be harmful or cause discomfort should be avoid. Now let's see what are the foods you should avoid and include in your diet.

Foods You Should Avoid in Your Diet

- **Irritating foods:** Vegetables such as tomatoes, garlic, onions, bell peppers and pickles; acidic or citrus fruits such as limes, lemons, oranges, pomegranate, grapefruit, tangerines, pineapple, passion fruit, cherries, plums, kiwis, green apples and grapes can irritate your stomach and worsen your symptoms of gastritis. Also avoid spices such as red or black pepper, curry, chili peppers, mint, and condiments such as ketchup, tomato sauce, vinegar, mustard, mayonnaise, hot sauces, salad dressings, and anything spicy or super salty.

- **Irritating drinks:** Coffee, alcoholic drinks, energy drinks, sodas or soft drinks, hot chocolate, strong teas (oolong, green or black tea), most herbal teas (most are too acidic to drink, try anise, fennel, ginger, licorice, or chamomile tea), all sugary drinks, and bottled juices with citric acid added. All these drinks can irritate the stomach lining and worsen the symptoms of gastritis.

- **Processed foods:** Avoid white or whole-grain bread, pastries, cookies, donuts, sponge cake, candy, chocolate, breakfast cereals, microwave popcorn, potato chips, fries, processed meats, sausages, instant soups, fast food, and everything processed. These are known as common inflammatory allergens that can trigger food allergies, increase inflammation in the intestines and slow down the healing process.

- **Dairy:** You may have heard that milk helps coat the stomach or neutralize stomach acid when you have stomach pain, but this advice is not entirely useful. Amino acids (protein) from milk stimulate stomach acid secretions, which can worsen the symptoms of gastritis. In addition, the protein in the cow, called beta-casein A1, is as inflammatory as —or even worse than— gluten. Therefore, it is advisable that you avoid dairy products and their derivatives, such as cheeses, whole and condensed milk, ice cream, yogurt, butter and custard desserts.

- **Bad fats:** High-fat foods slow down gastric emptying and increase inflammation in the stomach, so you will want to avoid deep-fried foods and processed foods made with saturated and trans fats. Some foods to avoid include hydrogenated or refined vegetable oils such as margarine, cream and butter, as well as commercial baked goods containing trans fats.

Foods You Should Include in Your Diet

- **Foods rich in flavonoids:** Vegetables such as spinach, broccoli, artichokes, asparagus, celery, kale, Brussels sprouts, okra and green leafy vegetables; fruits such as papaya, mangoes, apples (red delicious), peaches, berries, plums, cherries and apricots are all rich in flavonoids that help reduce inflammation and protect cells from the damage that free radicals cause. However, most fruits can be a little acidic for your stomach. It is advisable to eat low acid fruits (pH 5 or higher) such as papaya, melon, watermelon and bananas. One way to consume berries and some acidic fruits safely is through smoothies made with almond or another non-dairy milk to help neutralize their acidity.

- **Easy-to-digest foods:** Cooked vegetables and skinless fruits are on the list of easily digestible foods. Others to consider include white rice, instant oatmeal, white fish, skinless chicken or turkey, potatoes, carrots, sweet potatoes, squashes, and zucchini. Always choose soft-consistency and cooked foods instead of raw and hard foods, which cause mechanical irritation. Cooked foods are easier to digest, so you should steam, boil, bake or griddle your food.

- **High-quality proteins:** Lean proteins help repair the gastrointestinal wall and treat digestive problems such as intestinal permeability. Choose an easy-to-digest powdered protein such as hemp, pea or sprouted rice grains, as these are easier to assimilate and should not aggravate gastritis. Avoid protein derived from whey, as it is made from dairy and can worsen your symptoms. It is advisable that you eat organic eggs, organic chicken or turkey and wild-caught fish, and avoid all red meats as they are hard to digest.

- **Healthy fats:** Fat is an important nutrient that should be part of the diet to treat gastritis but only consumed in reasonable amounts. There are bad fats (trans and saturated) and good fats (polyunsaturated and monounsaturated), which are found mainly in avocados, nuts (walnuts, pecans, cashews, etc.), seeds (flaxseed, chia, hemp, etc.), cold-pressed vegetable oils such as olive oil, coconut oil, linseed oil, hemp oil, avocado oil and fishes such as salmon and sardines. It is advisable to include in your diet foods rich in Omega 3 (salmon, walnuts, chia and flaxseeds), as the essential fatty acids they contain help reduce inflammation. Limit your fat intake to a tablespoon of nuts or oil per meal.

- **Probiotics:** Introduce fermented foods and probiotics into your diet to improve intestinal health and reduce or prevent infections like that caused by *Helicobacter pylori*, which can contribute to gastritis. Although probiotics are generally found in milk and dairy (such as yogurt, cheese, whey, milk kefir, etc.), we can also find probiotics in fermented sauerkraut, miso, tempeh, non-dairy yogurt, and probiotic drinks such as kombucha and water kefir.

- **Fiber-rich foods:** Some scientific studies have shown that a diet rich in soluble fiber may be beneficial for gastritis and other digestive disorders, as mucilage protects and softens the stomach lining. Some of the best sources of soluble fiber include seeds such as chia and linseed; cereals such as oats or oat bran; fruits such as apples, mangoes, peaches and plums; and vegetables such as broccoli, Brussels sprouts, beets, eggplant, artichokes, asparagus, carrots, spinach, and okra.

General Recommendations

- **Manage your stress levels:** It is important that you reduce stress in your life, as it can worse gastritis and eventually trigger other health problems. Also, do not eat if you are stressed, as stress reduces the production of gastric juices and slow down digestion. Try to relax and be in a quiet atmosphere at lunch time. Learn to relax using relaxation techniques such as deep breathing, yoga, meditation, etc. A natural alternative to antidepressants drugs is an adaptogenic herb called Rhodiola rosea. This herb helps the body adapt to daily stress. It also decreases anxiety, depression, fatigue, and regulates cortisol levels.

- **Eat small meals:** Instead of eating three large meals a day, eat smaller meals more often. (You can split them into five or six meals.) Doing this can help increase blood flow to the stomach, which speeds up the healing process. On the other hand, large meals remain in the stomach for a long time and can significantly worsen symptoms. That's why it's best to eat no more than 1 cup of vegetables, 1 cup of rice, potatoes or another carbohydrate, and a portion of chicken breast or fish the size of your palm.

- **Chew food well:** Chew your food well and eat slowly, as this facilitates digestion and ensures that the stomach does not produce too much gastric juices to break down the food. It is advisable that you chew food three to five times more than normal or until they are practically liquified in your mouth.

- **Avoid drinking liquids with meals:** When you drink a lot of water or any liquid with meals, you dilute your gastric juices. Therefore, your stomach must expend more energy and nutrients to produce the gastric juices that digest food in the stomach. It is advisable that you drink water 30 minutes before and two hours after eating.
- **Do not lie down after eating:** For digestion to be carried out properly, you must be in an upright position. At bedtime, you compromise digestion. In addition, gastric juices may enter the esophagus and cause heartburn. Wait at least three hours before you lie down and raise the head of your bed about five or ten inches to avoid acid reflux.
- **Do not use anti-inflammatories drugs:** As you know, these types of drugs can damage the stomach lining, so you should avoid them. If you need analgesics, use acetaminophen.
- **Stay hydrated:** Drink as much water as you can daily to stay hydrated (aim to 2 liters), and try to drink a full glass of alkaline water when you feel the symptoms are getting worse. Coconut water is an excellent choice to increase hydration, cleanse the body of inflammation and provide electrolytes.
- **Exercise daily:** Exercise helps your body stay healthy and also stimulates the digestive system, which can help treat some of the symptoms of gastritis. Aerobic activities such as walking or jogging keep your digestive system moving regularly because they help the intestinal muscles work more efficiently. I recommend that you start walking for 20 to 30 minutes every day, preferably after eating, as this will help with the digestion process.

- **Reduce your sugar intake:** Sugar feeds bad bacteria and yeast like candida that damage your gut. Bad bacteria actually create toxins called exotoxins that damage healthy cells and cause leaky gut syndrome. If you are going to use a sweetener, use a moderate amount of coconut sugar, maple syrup, monk fruit or stevia. Avoid refined sugars and artificial sweeteners.

- **Do not smoke:** Cigarette/tobacco smoke irritates the esophagus and stomach lining, which can worsen gastritis symptoms. Smoking restricts the small blood vessels of the stomach, which reduces blood flow in the area and slows down the healing process.

- **Reduce your salt intake:** It is recommended that you reduce your salt intake and replace common table salt with a quality salt such as Himalayan or Celtic salt. Himalayan salt contains trace minerals that aid in the recovery process and support your body's overall health.

- **Take note of foods you cannot tolerate:** Every person with gastritis reacts differently to certain foods, so it is best to keep a diary of what you eat and identify those foods that make you feel bad. These are foods you should avoid for a while (several weeks); then reintroduce them one by one to see if the symptoms worsen. This way you will know whether you should avoid them for a long time so that you can control your symptoms and facilitate the healing process.

- **Consider using a gastroprotective agent:** Diet alone may not be enough to cure or improve stomach inflammation. Thus, it is recommended that you use a gastroprotective drug such as sucralfate, which protects the stomach lining from the irritating action of stomach acid and pepsin. Consult your doctor for a prescription for this drug.

- **Tips to gaining weight:** If you need to gain weight, you must consume more calories. Fat contains the most calories (9 calories per gram), followed by carbohydrates and proteins (4 calories per gram). If you want to gain weight, eat more carbohydrates (such as white rice, sweet potatoes, squashes, etc.) and fats, bearing in mind that too much fat (regardless of whether it is good or bad) slows down gastric emptying and can increases inflammation. Try adding a little fat in reasonable amounts — for example, a handful of walnuts in oatmeal, a tablespoon of olive oil or half a small avocado at each meal.

Other recommendations include eating foods at room temperature and avoiding foods or drinks that are very hot or cold; and avoiding foods with gluten or wheat. Also make sure you get enough sleep to help with the recovery process.

CHAPTER 5

SUPPLEMENTS AND REMEDIES

Several natural remedies and supplements can help reduce stomach inflammation and the symptoms related to gastritis. Therefore, include in your therapeutic regimen some of the supplements and natural remedies mentioned below.

Supplements for Gastritis

Slippery Elm

The inner bark of the Ulmus rubra tree creates a mucilaginous protective layer around the stomach lining, protecting it from stomach acid and relieving the symptoms of gastritis. Slippery elm is available in capsules and powder; take two capsules between meals with a glass of water, or mix a teaspoon of slippery elm powder with a glass of water or juice.

L-Glutamine

This is the most abundant amino acid in the body. It helps improve gastrointestinal health, as it is a vital nutrient for the intestines and assists in the repair of damaged tissues. Glutamine can help decrease inflammation and stomach damage caused by *Helicobacter pylori*. It is advised that you take 5 to 10 grams of glutamine daily (divided into two shots) on an empty stomach or dilute 4 teaspoons in a liter bottle of water and sip it throughout the day.

DGL (Deglycyrrhizinated Licorice)

This is the root of the plant Glycyrrhiza glabra, which is known for its antispasmodic, anti-inflammatory and protective properties to the stomach lining. Various scientific studies have shown that licorice helps heal duodenal and gastric ulcers. It acts by forming a layer on the mucosa of the stomach, protecting it from the corrosive action of the gastric juices and favoring their healing. You can find it in chewable tablets or powder form. Take the dose as directed by the manufacturer.

Probiotics

Probiotics help boost the number of beneficial microorganisms in the digestive tract and help fight opportunistic bacteria such as *Helicobacter pylori*, which damage the digestive tract. Some of the most common species of probiotics are Lactobacillus and Bifidobacterium, which colonize the lining of the intestinal tract and boost the digestive system's ability to digest food and absorb nutrients. Consider taking a probiotic containing 10 to 50 billion CFUs before breakfast or after dinner. You can also include probiotic drinks such as kefir or kombucha.

Gamma-oryzanol

This supplement is obtained from rice bran, which is on the outer covering of the grain of this cereal. Gamma-oryzanol is a complex formed by the mixture of plant sterols and ferulic acid (a natural antioxidant), which helps protect the stomach lining; thus, it is indicated in cases of gastritis or gastric ulcers. You can find it in capsules or tablets. Take the dose indicated by the manufacturer.

Zinc

This mineral, which is also an antioxidant, is necessary for stimulating a catalytic enzyme called carbonic anhydrase. Without this enzyme, your stomach cannot produce bicarbonate or stomach acid. The bicarbonate combines with the gastric mucus and acts as a buffer against stomach acid to prevent self-digestion of the stomach lining. Although zinc deficiency is common, it is recommended that you consult with a physician before you start taking this supplement.

Zinc Carnosine

This is a complex of zinc and the amino acid L-carnosine, which is also a potent antioxidant. This supplement helps protect the stomach lining from opportunistic bacteria such as *Helicobacter pylori* and NSAID (non-steroidal anti-inflammatory drug) damage. It also supports the health of gastric cells and has gastroprotective properties. Take two capsules (about 75mg) of zinc carnosine two times daily with meal.

Omega 3

Omega-3 fatty acids, such as fish oil, have anti-inflammatory properties that help reduce the severity of symptoms and promote healing. The best source of omega-3 is krill oil because it contains a powerful antioxidant and anti-inflammatory carotenoid called astaxanthin, as well as phospholipids that increase the absorption of their fats. The recommended dose is one or two capsules or 1 tablespoon of omega-3-rich oil two to three times a day or as directed by the manufacturer.

Vitamin A

This vitamin is an essential antioxidant for maintaining the mucous membranes of the stomach lining in healthy conditions. Take 3,000 to 5,000 IU of vitamin A every day.

Also consider taking a good food-based or low-acid multivitamin supplement. Nutritional deficiencies are common in people suffering from gastrointestinal disorders such as gastritis or leaky gut, and even in those who follow a "healthy diet."

Natural Remedies for Gastritis

Potato Juice

Another effective remedy for gastritis is raw potato juice, due to its antacid and healing properties. The alkaline properties of potatoes help reduce swelling, relieve the pain of stomach ulcers and calm stomach upset. Some studies have shown that starch from the potato extract attaches to the injured stomach lining and provides a protective barrier effect against stomach acid.

Ingredients:
- 1 or 2 large red potatoes

Directions:
1. Wash the potatoes well and then peel them.
2. Place the peeled potatoes in a juice extractor to extract the juice.
3. Drink it immediately. (Do not let the starch sit on the bottom of the glass.)

Notes
- Never use potatoes that are not ripe (green) or potatoes with black dots, as potatoes contain high concentrations of a toxic substance called solanine.
- You can drink the potato juice one to three times a day, half an hour before each meal. If the taste is not pleasant, combine the potato juice with fresh carrot juice; this increases its healing properties.

Aloe Vera

Aloe vera is a medicinal plant that has been used for centuries and is known for its anti-inflammatory and healing properties on the skin and mucous membranes. The gel inside this plant contains a compound called mucilage that, thanks to its viscous texture, protects the stomach lining and favors its regeneration. This is beneficial for treating ulcers and gastritis.

Ingredients:
- 1 aloe vera leaf

Directions:
1. With a knife, cut the rows of thorns from the sides of the aloe vera leaf.
2. Wash the aloe vera leaf.
3. Cut the leaf into pieces approximately 2 inches long and let soak for 24 hours, changing the water every four or six hours.
4. Then, with a knife, remove the green outer layer and place the gel in an airtight container.
5. Chew about 2 or 3 tablespoons of the aloe vera gel on an empty stomach.

Notes
- It is important to take this remedy in the right way to relieve the symptoms associated with gastritis. It is recommended that you chew (on an empty stomach)

three tablespoons of freshly extracted aloe vera gel. Thus, mucilage can act directly on irritated or inflamed stomach lining. You should take this remedy 30 minutes before eating or two or three hours after eating about three times a day.

- You can also mix 16 ounces of aloe juice with 16 ounces or more of water and sip on it throughout the day. Do this for two months, then wean down to 8 ounces of juice for another month.

Chamomile Tea

The chamomile flower is rich in certain essential oils that are beneficial in repairing the stomach lining. This herb contains high levels of apigenin, a flavonoid that reduces inflammation. It also contains a component called Bisabolol, which seems to be primarily responsible for its anti-inflammatory and reparative properties to the digestive system.

Ingredients:

- 1 tablespoon of chamomile flowers (or one sachet)
- 1 cup water
- Maple syrup, to taste (optional)

Directions:

1. Heat a cup of water. When it is boiling, turn off the heat.
2. Pour the chamomile flowers into warm water, cover with a lid (so that the essential oils do not escape) and let stand for 15 minutes.
3. Strain (after 15 minutes) and cool. Drink it immediately.

Note

- It is recommended that you take this tea at least three times a day. Remember that you should not boil this herb because high temperatures can destroy its active compounds.

Ginger Tea

Ginger can effectively treat gastritis because of its anti-inflammatory and antibacterial properties. A research concluded that gingerol compounds significantly inhibited the growth of *Helicobacter pylori*, a bacterium associated with many stomach problems, including gastritis and gastroduodenal ulcers.

Ingredients:

- 1 slice fresh ginger, peeled (about 20 grams)
- 1 cup water
- Maple syrup, to taste (optional)

Directions:

1. Wash the piece of ginger well and cut into small pieces.
2. Heat the cup of water. When it is boiling, turn off the heat.
3. Pour the chopped ginger into the pan containing the hot water and let sit for 10 minutes over low heat.
4. Turn off the heat. Wait another five minutes and use a strainer to remove the chopped ginger before serving. Drink it 20 minutes before eating, once or twice a day.

Note

- Ginger may interfere with anticoagulant medications and high blood pressure.

Bone Broth

Broth is a mineral-rich infusion made by boiling the bones of healthy animals with vegetables and herbs. Bone broth is great for healing intestinal permeability (leaky gut) and reducing gut inflammation. You can drink a cup of bone broth every day to help heal the stomach lining.

Ingredients:

- 4 pounds Chicken necks/feet/wings (preferibly organic)
- 3 Carrots, chopped
- 3 Celery Stalks, chopped
- ½ cup Fresh Parsley and Dill leaves
- 20 cups Cold Water
- 2 Kale leaves
- 1 teaspoon Himalayan or Celtic salt
- 3 tablespoons Organic Apple Cider Vinegar

Directions:

1. Place all ingredients in a 10-quart-capacity crock pot.
2. Add the water. Simmer for 24-48 hours, skimming fat occasionally.
3. Remove from heat and allow to cool slightly. Discard solids and strain the remainder in a bowl through a colander. Let stock cool to room temperature, cover and chill.
4. Use within a week or freeze for up to three months.

Note

- You can increase the broth's gut-healing properties by adding three or five grams of L-glutamine to a cup of bone broth before drinking it.

PART THREE

THE RECIPES

CHAPTER 6

BREAKFAST RECIPES

SIMPLE OATMEAL

This is a healthy and excellent breakfast to start the day. Oatmeal provides the benefits of soluble fiber that helps improve gut flora and prevent constipation.

SERVINGS 2 | **PREP TIME** 5 MINS | **COOK TIME** 12 MINS

1 cup Water
1 cup Almond Milk
1 cup Gluten Free Instant Oats
1 ripe Banana, sliced
1-2 tablespoons Unsweetened Coconut Flakes or Chopped Walnuts (optional)
Maple Syrup, to taste (optional)

Directions

1. In a nonstick pan, add oats and cook by stirring continuously for about 4-6 minutes on medium heat. Add water and reduce the heat to medium-low.

2. Add almond milk and cook for about 6 to 8 minutes or until the liquid is absorbed.

3. Serve with sliced banana and coconut flakes and/or maple syrup on top.

BLUEBERRY BANANA SMOOTHIE BOWL

A creamy bowl of banana and blueberries. Similar in texture to soft serve ice cream topped with crunchy granola.

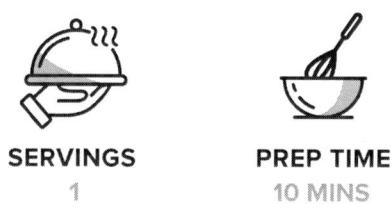

SERVINGS	PREP TIME	COOK TIME
1	10 MINS	N/A

1 or 2 Frozen Bananas
½ cup Frozen Blueberries
½ cup Almond Milk
1 tablespoon Almond Butter
Maple Syrup, to taste
Granola (optional)

Directions

1. Add all the ingredients in a blender and blend until thick and creamy.
2. Pour into a medium bowl and top with granola of your choice (if using).
3. Serve immediately and enjoy!

SPINACH MUSHROOM SCRAMBLED EGGS

This classic recipe is easy to make and ideal for breakfast. Both spinach and eggs are packed with nutrients your body needs.

SERVINGS
1

PREP TIME
5 MINS

COOK TIME
8 MINS

1 Egg + 2 Egg Whites
¼ cup Fresh Mushrooms, sliced
½ cup Fresh Spinach, trimmed and chopped finely
Olive Oil Cooking Spray, as required
Pinch of Fresh Parsley, minced (optional)
Pinch of Salt

Directions

1. In a bowl, add the spinach, eggs, and salt and beat lightly.
2. Coat a nonstick pan with cooking oil spray and put on medium heat. Add mushrooms; cook and stir 3-5 minutes or until tender.
3. Add egg mixture and cook for 4 to 5 minutes or until set completely.
4. Garnish with parsley (optional). Serve and enjoy!

PUMPKIN SPINACH SMOOTHIE

A healthy and creamy green smoothie loaded with vitamins, minerals and antioxidants from pumpkin, banana and spinach. Autumn never tasted so delicious!

SERVINGS	PREP TIME	COOK TIME
1	5 MINS	N/A

1 Frozen Ripe Banana
¼ cup Pumpkin Purée
¼ cup Light Coconut Milk
⅓ cup Unsweetened Almond Milk
1 cup Fresh Spinach

Directions

1. Place all ingredients to a blender and blend until smooth and creamy, scraping down sides as needed. If too thick, add more almond or coconut milk.
2. Taste and adjust flavor as needed. For more sweetness, add more banana or a bit of maple syrup or honey.
3. Serve immediately. Best when fresh, though will keep in the refrigerator well covered up to 1-2 days.

BUCKWHEAT WAFFLES

These delicious Belgian waffles made with buckwheat flour are crispy on the outside and light on the inside. A great recipe for breakfast or brunch.

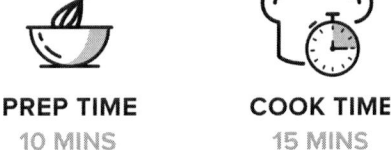

SERVINGS
6 WAFFLES

PREP TIME
10 MINS

COOK TIME
15 MINS

2 large Eggs, separated
2 cups Buckwheat Flour
4 teaspoons Baking Powder
½ tablespoon Coconut Sugar
1 ¾ cups Unsweetened Almond Milk
3 tablespons Coconut Oil, melted
½ teaspoon Vanilla Extract
¼ teaspoon Salt

Directions

1. Prepare waffle iron with cooking spray and turn it on to warm it. (As you continue to make all of the waffles, be sure to spray the waffle iron each time with cooking spray. These waffles will stick, if you don't.)
2. Separate egg yolks from egg whites. It is important to try to keep all of the egg yolks out of your egg whites. Set egg whites aside.

3. Use a mixer to beat all ingredients (including egg yolks) together, except egg whites. Transfer mixture to a large bowl (unless you have more than one mixer). Clean the mixing bowl and beaters.
4. Beat egg whites at a high speed for about 4 minutes and until soft peaks have formed. Stir egg whites into the waffle batter.
5. Use a ½ cup measuring cup to spoon mixture out and onto waffle iron. (This amount may vary depending on the size of your waffle iron). Close the waffle iron and cook until the waffles are barely letting off steam and they are lightly crisp to the touch (this might take longer than your waffle maker suggests). Repeat with remaining batter as necessary.
6. Serve with toppings of your choice (maple syrup, almond butter and/or sliced banana) and enjoy!

Note

- These waffles store well in the freezer. Re-heat them in the oven at 300 degrees F for a couple of minutes.

BLUEBERRY ALMOND SMOOTHIE

A delicious and perfect smoothie to start the morning loaded with antioxidants, fiber and healthy fats.

SERVINGS	PREP TIME	COOK TIME
2	5 MINS	N/A

½ cup Frozen Blueberries
1 Frozen Ripe Banana
1 cup Unsweetened Almond Milk
½ tablespoon Almond Butter
1 tablespoon Flaxseed Meal
1 tablespoon Chia Seeds

Directions

1. Add frozen banana, blueberries, almond butter, chia seeds, flaxseed meal, and almond milk to a blender and blend on high speed until creamy and smooth.
2. Serve immediately and enjoy!

Note

- Add a bit more almond milk if your blender has trouble blending. Then taste and adjust flavor as needed, adding more banana (or a bit of honey) for sweetness, almond butter for creaminess, blueberries for fruitiness, or almond milk to thin.

CHIA RICE PUDDING

An easy to make and digest pudding, very comforting and ideal for those moments when your tummy feels bad.

SERVINGS 2
PREP TIME 5 MINS
COOK TIME 30 MINS

2 cups Almond Milk
½ cup Uncooked White Rice
1 tablespoon Coconut Sugar
½ teaspoon Vanilla Extract
1 tablespoon Raisins (optional)
2 tablespoons Chia Seeds

Directions

1. Place the milk, sugar and rice in a medium saucepan and bring to a boil over medium-high heat, stirring occasionally until the sugar has dissolved.
2. Lower the heat to a simmer and cook uncovered, stirring occasionally, until the rice is tender and the mixture thickens, about 20 minutes.
3. Remove from the heat and stir in the vanilla extract. Allow to cool to room temperature, stirring 1-2 times to break up the chia and prevent clumping. Once cool, cover and refrigerate overnight. To serve, stir the chilled pudding and top with raisins, if desired. Enjoy!

BANANA OAT PANCAKES

These fluffy banana pancakes are ideal for those lazy mornings. Serve with fresh fruits and other toppings.

SERVINGS	PREP TIME	COOK TIME
2	10 MINS	15 MINS

½ medium Banana
¾ cup Gluten Free Rolled Oats (or oat flour)
½ cup Almond Milk
1 teaspoon Baking Powder
1 tablespoon Maple Syrup
Pinch of Salt
Olive Oil for greasing

Directions

1. Heat a pan on medium heat. Add olive oil to grease the pan.
2. Pulse the rolled oats in a food processor until fine flour forms. (Alternatively use a blender or beater) If using oat flour, add to food processor.
3. Once oats are ground, add in the banana, milk, and baking powder and pulse again until smooth batter forms. If you're using oat flour you can use a hand-held blender to beat batter (a whisk will also work).
4. Using ¼ cup measuring cup add pancake batter to prepared pan and cook 2-3 minutes before flipping. Cook additional 2 minutes on other side. Serve and enjoy!

STEWED APPLES & BLUEBERRIES

A light and simple breakfast of cooked apples loaded with antioxidants to help fight free-radicals and increase vitality.

SERVINGS
1

PREP TIME
10 MINS

COOK TIME
25 MINS

2 Red Apples
½ cup Coconut or Almond Milk
A handful of Blueberries
½ inch Fresh Ginger, grated
1 teaspoon Maple Syrup
Granola (optional)

Directions

1. Peel, core and dice the apples and place them in a saucepan with the coconut or almond milk, blueberries, maple syrup, and ginger.
2. Cook the mixture on a medium-heat until it begins to boil, reduce the heat if needs be but keep it simmering for about 15-20 minutes until the apples are soft and part of the liquid has been absorbed. Add more milk or water if needed.
3. Serve topped with granola (optional). Enjoy!

FRENCH TOAST

A moist, slightly sweet and tasty bread high in egg protein. This is an excellent gluten-free French toast bread recipe.

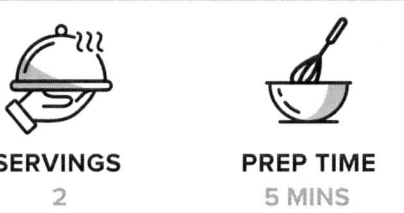

SERVINGS
2

PREP TIME
5 MINS

COOK TIME
10 MINS

1 large Egg, beaten
¼ - ⅓ cup Coconut Milk
4 slices Gluten Free Bread
½ teaspoon Coconut Sugar
½ teaspoon Vanilla Extract
Pinch of Salt (optional)
Olive Oil for greasing

Directions

1. Combine the egg, milk, vanilla, sugar and salt in a mixing bowl and whisk until thoroughly blended.
2. Dunk each of the bread slices in the egg mixture. Allow each slice of bread to soak up as much egg mixture as it will hold.
3. Heat oil over medium-high in a large skillet and cook the coated bread slices. When golden brown, flip and cook second side until golden brown.
4. Serve warm with maple syrup (or toppings of your choice on top) and enjoy.

RICE PORRIDGE

This rice porridge is delicious on its own, but even better with a sliced banana or some blueberries in the mix.

SERVINGS
2

PREP TIME
5 MINS

COOK TIME
10 MINS

1 cup Almond Milk
1 cup Cooked White Rice
1 Sliced Banana or ½ cup Blueberries
1 tablespoon Chia Seeds or Flaxseed Meal (optional)
1 tablespoon Maple Syrup
Pinch of Salt

Directions

1. Put the cup of the pre-cooked rice in a small pot on a low heat, add the almond milk and chia seeds or flaxseed meal (if using) and allow to simmer for 5-8 minutes until all ingredients are soft.
2. Serve and top with blueberries or a sliced banana and maple syrup.

COCONUT FLOUR PUMPKIN PANCAKES

This recipe delivers light and fluffy pancakes that are perfect for your leisurely Saturday or Sunday mornings.

SERVINGS
6 PANCAKES

PREP TIME
5 MINS

COOK TIME
10 MINS

2 large Eggs
½ cup Pumpkin Purée
⅓ cup Coconut Flour
½ cup Unsweetened Almond or Coconut Milk
½ teaspoon Vanilla Extract
1 tablespoon Maple Syrup
½ teaspoon Baking Soda
Coconut oil for greasing
¼ teaspoon Salt

Directions

1. Preheat griddle or a large skillet over medium heat and grease with the oil.
2. In a large mixing bowl, combine the pumpkin, eggs, milk, maple syrup and vanilla. Mix well to combine.
3. In a separate smaller bowl, combine the coconut flour, baking soda and salt.
4. Slowly add the flour mixture into the bowl of the wet

mixture, stirring continuously, and mix until completely combined. Do not over mix.
5. Place ¼ cup of the batter on the pre-heated griddle or large skillet to form a pancake. Cook during 4-5 minutes or until pancakes begin to bubble in the center. Then flip and cook another 2-4 minutes on the other side until lightly browned.
6. Transfer pancakes to a cooling rack and repeat the process with the remaining batter.
7. Serve and top with desired toppings and enjoy!

APPLE PIE QUINOA PORRIDGE

Quinoa takes the place of oats and makes this a healthy and nutritious breakfast. It really do tastes like you are eating apple pie for breakfast!

SERVINGS
4

PREP TIME
10 MINS

COOK TIME
15 MINS

1 cup Quinoa, rinsed
¼ cup Unsweetened Applesauce
2 cups Unsweetened Almond Milk
¼ teaspoon Vanilla Extract
2 medium Red Apples, shredded
Maple Syrup (optional)
Pinch of Salt

Directions

1. In a medium saucepan, bring the almond milk, quinoa and applesauce to a boil.
2. Once the quinoa starts to boil, reduce to a simmer and cook covered for 15 minutes until most of the liquid is absorbed. Stir in the vanilla and salt.
3. Pour the quinoa porridge into bowls and top with shredded apples and a drizzle of maple syrup if desired.
4. Cover and refrigerate leftovers.

RICE BANANA WAFFLES

This is a simple waffle recipe made with rice and banana. It's a perfect fuel for a delicious weekend breakfast.

SERVINGS 3 **PREP TIME** 10 MINS **COOK TIME** 10 MINS

2 Eggs
2 cups Cooked White Rice
1 medium Banana
1 tablespoon Coconut Oil
1 tablespoon Coconut Sugar
½ teaspoon Baking Powder
1 tablespoon Tapioca Flour or Potato Flour
½ cup Almond or Coconut Milk
1 teaspoon Vanilla Extract
Pinch of Salt

Directions

1. Place all ingredients (except the milk) in a blender and pulse until mixed, then turn on low and add the milk. Blend until smooth and thick. Keep the mixture in the blender.
2. Preheat a waffle iron and grease with oil.
3. Pour the mixture onto the preheated waffle iron. Cook until golden brown, around 6-10 minutes per waffle.
4. Remove from the waffle iron and serve warm or let cool then wrap in foil and place in freezer for later.

BANANA CHIA SEED CUSTARD

This banana chia custard recipe is light and tasty. Definitely a winner on those warm summery nights and a perfect choice when you need a quick and satisfying breakfast.

SERVINGS
2

PREP TIME
5 MINS

COOK TIME
5 MINS

2 Egg Yolks
1 Banana, sliced
1 can (13.5 oz) Coconut Milk
1 tablespoon Vanilla Extract
¼ cup Chia Seeds
¼ teaspoon Salt
4-6 Dates

Directions

1. Pour the coconut milk into a saucepan and heat over medium-high heat. Place the egg yolks in a bowl.
2. Once the coconut milk starts to scald, slowly pour about one cup of the hot milk into the egg yolks, stirring continuously, with a whisk.
3. Add the milk/egg mixture back to the saucepan and heat over medium heat for about 4-5 minutes, stirring constantly. The mixture should thicken slightly, do not boil.

4. Pour the mixture into a blender and add the banana, dates, vanilla and salt. Blend on high speed to combine for 2-3 minutes, until smooth. Add the chia seeds and pulse to evenly combine. Pour the mixture into 4 ramekins or small jars.
5. Cover and refrigerate overnight. Serve topped with banana slices and walnuts and enjoy!!

Note

- To make this recipe egg-free simply omit the egg yolks and blend all the ingredients in the blender.

SWEET POTATO PANCAKES

Sweet potato adds a rich creaminess to these pancakes which are delicious served with maple syrup.

SERVINGS
6 PANCAKES

PREP TIME
10 MINS

COOK TIME
20 MINS

2 Eggs
⅓ cup Coconut Flour
1 tablespoon Coconut Sugar
1 teaspoon Baking Powder
½ cup Cooked Sweet Potato, mashed
½ cup Unsweetened Almond Milk
1 tablespoon Coconut Oil, melted
½ teaspoon Vanilla Extract
½ teaspoon Salt

Directions

1. In a medium mixing bowl, combine coconut flour, coconut sugar, baking powder and salt.
2. In a large bowl, whisk together almond milk, coconut oil, eggs, vanilla and mashed sweet potatoes. (You can use a blender or a immersion blender).
3. Pour the dry mixture into the large bowl with wet ingredients. Stir to combine. (If too thick, add more almond milk).

4. Preheat a nonstick skillet over medium heat and grease with oil. Ladle about 2-3 tablespoons of the batter and cook for about 3 minutes, flip, and continue cooking for another 3 minutes on the other side or until pancake is firm and slightly golden brown. Continue with the remaining batter.
5. Serve and top with desired toppings and enjoy!

Note

- Leftovers can be store in the fridge in a glass container for up to 1 week.

COCONUT BREAD

Coconut flour bread is one of the easiest and healthiest recipe. This recipe is loaded with protein, healthy fats and prebiotic fiber which is great for maintaining a healthy digestive system.

SERVINGS
10 SLICES

PREP TIME
10 MINS

COOK TIME
30 MINS

2 Eggs + 3 Egg Whites
½ cup Coconut Flour
½ cup Buckwheat Flour
½ cup canned Coconut Milk
2 tablespoons Coconut Oil
1 teaspoon Baking Powder
1 teaspoon Liquid Stevia or 4 tbsp. Coconut Sugar
½ teaspoon Salt

Directions

1. In a medium mixing bowl, combine the eggs, coconut oil, stevia and salt. Add the coconut milk and mix well.
2. Add the buckwheat flour, coconut flour and baking powder, and whisk until you don't see any lumps.
3. Pour the mixture into a 8x4 inch loaf pan greased with coconut oil and bake at 175°C (350 degrees F) for about 30 minutes.
4. Remove the bread from the oven and allow it to cool. (The top of the loaf should be firm and a light golden brown).

BANANA BREAD

A hybrid between banana bread and a drizzle cake. This banana loaf recipe is easy to make, and does not take much time for its preparation.

SERVINGS 10 SLICES   **PREP TIME** 10 MINS   **COOK TIME** 60 MINS

3 medium Bananas (1 cup aprox.)
¼ cup Almond or Coconut Milk
⅓ cup Coconut Oil, melted
1 tablespoon Coconut Sugar
2 cups Gluten Free Flour
1 teaspoon Baking Powder
1 teaspoon Baking Soda
¼ teaspoon Salt

Directions

1. Preheat oven to 350 degrees F (175°C). Grease a 9x5 inch loaf pan, set aside.
2. In a large mixing bowl, combine the flour, baking powder, baking soda and salt, set aside. In a small bowl, mix coconut oil and sugar. Stir in milk.
3. Mash bananas and combine with wet ingredients. Stir banana mixture into flour mixture; stir until well combined. Pour mixture into the prepared loaf pan.
4. Bake in preheated oven for 50 to 60 minutes, until a toothpick inserted into center of the loaf comes out clean.
5. Let bread cool in pan for at least 10 minutes, then remove onto a wire rack. Slice and serve warm!

BUCKWHEAT & QUINOA PORRIDGE

A creamy buckwheat porridge made with healthy ingredients such as almond milk, chia seeds and quinoa which make this a nutritious breakfast.

SERVINGS
2

PREP TIME
5 MINS

COOK TIME
20 MINS

3 cup Water
⅓ cup Quinoa
2 cup Almond Milk
½ cup hulled Buckwheat Groats
1 tablespoon Coconut Oil
1 tablespoon Maple Syrup
⅓ cup Chia Seeds

Directions

1. In a large saucepan on medium heat, melt coconut oil.
2. Rinse quinoa in strainer. Toast quinoa and buckwheat on medium heat for 3-5 minutes, making sure to stir so that all seeds are coated with coconut oil.
3. Add water and turn heat on high heat. Bring to a boil, cover and turn down to medium-low heat. Cook covered, at a simmer, for about 20 minutes.
4. In a medium bowl, whisk maple syrup into almond milk.

5. Remove lid from saucepan. Stir in milk and add chia seeds. Add an additional cup of milk, if you desire a thinner consistency. (Chia seeds will absorb most of the excess liquid and the porridge will become thicker after sitting for about 10 minutes.).
6. Serve and top with nuts of your choice and a few fresh or frozen blueberries (optional).

Note

- Leftovers keep in fridge for 2-3 days for freshest taste.

BLUEBERRY MUFFINS

These fluffy and healthy low-fat muffins are delicious and easy to make. Try them for breakfast or brunch.

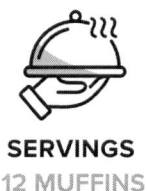

SERVINGS	PREP TIME	COOK TIME
12 MUFFINS	10 MINS	25 MINS

1 ½ cups Blueberries
3 cups Gluten Free All-Purpose Flour
½ cup Applesauce or Mashed Bananas
1 ½ cups Unsweetened Almond Milk
4 tablespoons Coconut Sugar
4 teaspoons Baking Powder
1 teaspoon Vanilla Extract
¼ teaspoon Salt

Directions

1. Preheat the oven to 400 degrees F. Lightly grease and line a 12-count muffin tin with muffin liners.
2. In a large bowl, combine the flour, sugar, baking powder and salt until well combined.
3. Add the applesauce or mashed bananas, almond milk, and vanilla to the dry ingredients and mix well. Fold in the blueberries.
4. Evenly distribute the muffin mixture amongst the 12

muffin liners and bake in the oven for 25-30 minutes, or until a toothpick inserted into the center comes out clean.
5. Once cooked, remove from oven and allow in the pan for 10 minutes, and then remove from pan and let cool completely on a cooling rack.

BLUEBERRY CHIA PUDDING

A healthy breakfast on the go, loaded with fiber, protein, and antioxidants. Serve with toasted almonds and blueberries.

SERVINGS	PREP TIME	COOK TIME
2	10 MINS	N/A

½ cup Chia Seeds
½ cup Fresh Blueberries
2 cups Unsweetened Almond Milk
¼ cup Toasted Slivered or Sliced Almonds
½ teaspoon Vanilla Extract
2 tablespoon Maple Syrup (optional)

Directions

1. Place the almond milk and blueberries in a blender and pulse until well combined. Pour the mixture into a bowl or a quart-sized mason jar.
2. Stir in the chia seeds, maple syrup, and vanilla. (Alternatively, and if using a mason jar, you can just cover and shake it well). Let sit for 10-15 minutes, then stir again to break up any clumping.
3. Place in the fridge for a minimum of 2 hours, or preferably overnight.
4. Top and serve as desired. Enjoy!

COCONUT QUINOA PORRIDGE

Supercharge your morning with this high-protein and creamy porridge topped with seasonal fruit

SERVINGS 2

PREP TIME 10 MINS

COOK TIME 15 MINS

½ cup Quinoa
2 ¼ cups Coconut Milk
1 teaspoon Vanilla Extract
1 tablespoon Maple Syrup
Chopped fruits (such as, banana or mango)
2 tablespoon Almonds, flaked (optional)
2 tablespoons Coconut Flakes

Directions

1. Rinse the quinoa and drain. Add to a medium saucepan with the coconut milk, maple syrup and vanilla. Bring to a boil.
2. Reduce the heat to a simmer for 15 minutes, until the quinoa has absorbed most of the liquid.
3. Pour the quinoa porridge between two bowls and stir in a little milk, to make it creamy.
4. Serve with the chopped fruits and coconut flakes or flaked almonds (if using). Enjoy!

BANANA CRUMBLE

This banana crumble has unique flavor and aroma that makes it great for breakfast or a dinner party dessert.

SERVINGS 2
PREP TIME 10 MINS
COOK TIME 10 MINS

1 large Banana, chopped into 1-inch pieces
1 tablespoon Almond Milk
1 teaspoon Vanilla Extract

Crumble topping

¼ cup Ground Almonds
¼ cup Desiccated Coconut
1 tablespoon Coconut Oil, melted
2 tablespoons Almond Milk

Directions

1. Preheat the oven to 180 degrees C.
2. Soften the bananas on a low heat on the hob with the almond milk and vanilla.
3. In a small bowl, mix together the ground almonds and desiccated coconut. Stir in the coconut oil. Then, add the almond milk and stir until the mixture clumps together.
4. Divide the banana mixture between two ramekin dishes.
5. Top with the crumble mixture and bake for about 10 minutes until the top turns crisp and golden brown.
6. Serve and enjoy!

TURKEY BREAKFAST SAUSAGE

A savory and easy to make recipe for turkey breakfast sausage patties that the entire family will love!

SERVINGS
4

PREP TIME
10 MINS

COOK TIME
15 MINS

12 ounces Ground Turkey Breast
1 tablespoon Ground Sage
½ teaspoon Dried Thyme
½ teaspoon Ground Fennel Seed
1 teaspoon Olive Oil
½ teaspoon Salt

Directions

1. In a medium bowl, combine the ground turkey, sage, thyme, fennel, and salt. Form the mixture into 8 patties.
2. Heat the oil in a nonstick skillet over medium-high heat. Once the oil shimmers, add the patties and cook until browned, about 4 minutes per side.

Note

- You can double or triple the batch and freeze the patties in zip-top freezer bags for use during the week. You just have thaw them in the refrigerator before reheating them.

COCONUT ALMOND CEREAL

This coconut crisps cereal is a healthier version of the sugar-laden breakfast cereals found in the supermarkets.

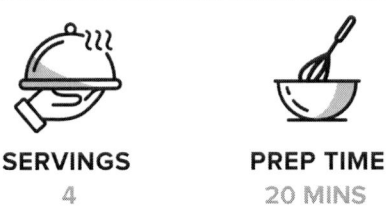

SERVINGS 4

PREP TIME 20 MINS

COOK TIME 12 MINS

1 Egg White
1 ½ cups Almond Flour
½ cup Unsweetened Shredded Coconut
1 tablespoon Coconut Oil, melted
¼ teaspoon Baking Soda
½ teaspoon Vanilla Extract
½ teaspoon Stevia Powder
¼ teaspoon Salt

Directions

1. Preheat oven to 350°F (177 degrees C).
2. Combine the almond flour, unsweetened shredded coconut, baking soda, and salt in a medium mixing bowl. Set aside.
3. Whisk melted coconut oil, stevia powder and vanilla in a small bowl.
4. In another small bowl, whisk egg white until frothy. Combine egg white and coconut oil mixture, whisk thoroughly.

5. Add wet ingredients to dry ingredients and stir until well combined.
6. Place the dough between two pieces of parchment paper and roll it out until it is 1/16 inch thick. Then remove the top piece of parchment paper.
7. Transfer the bottom piece of parchment paper with the rolled-out dough onto a baking sheet. With a knife or pizza cutter, cut the dough into 1-inch squares and bake for about 12 minutes.
8. Remove from the oven and let cool for 5 minutes, then serve with almond or coconut milk.

CHAPTER 7

POULTRY & SEAFOOD RECIPES

CHICKEN & VEGGIE STIR-FRY

This easy and tasty chicken stir-fry recipe is loaded with fresh veggies and a delicious sauce made with sesame oil, ginger, and coconut aminos.

SERVINGS
2

PREP TIME
20 MINS

COOK TIME
15 MINS

1 Boneless, Skinless Chicken Breast, cut into pieces
1 ½ cups Broccoli, cut into florets
1 medium Carrot, peeled and julienned
½ medium Zucchini, sliced
⅔ cup Mushrooms, sliced (optional)
1 tablespoon Olive or Coconut Oil
1 teaspoon Ginger, grated
3 tablespoons Coconut Aminos or Bragg Liquid Aminos
1 tablespoon Toasted Sesame Oil
1 teaspoon Arrowroot Flour or NON-GMO Cornstarch

Directions

1. In a large nonstick skillet or wok over medium-high heat, add the olive oil, ginger, and chicken, and cook, stirring occasionally, until the chicken is cooked or slightly browned. Remove the chicken from the skillet and set aside.

2. Add the vegetables to the skillet and cook, stirring frequently, until tender, about 5-8 minutes.
3. In a small mixing bowl, mix the coconut aminos or Bragg liquid aminos, sesame oil, and arrowroot flour or cornstarch.
4. Add the chicken back to the skillet and pour the stir-fry sauce on top. Stir well and simmer, stirring occasionally, for an additional 2 to 3 minutes. Serve and enjoy.

GRILLED SALMON WITH YOGURT SAUCE

This grilled salmon with yogurt is not only tasty and healthy, it is also an excellent choice for those who like yogurt but follow a dairy-free diet.

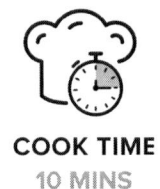

SERVINGS
2

PREP TIME
15 MINS

COOK TIME
10 MINS

2 (4-ounces) Salmon Fillets
2 tablespoons Non-Dairy Yogurt
1 teaspoon Extra Virgin Olive Oil
2 tablespoons Fresh Thyme, chopped
2 tablespoons Fresh Rosemary, chopped
½ teaspoon Freshly Ground Cumin
Salt, to taste

Directions

1. Combine all of the ingredients (except the salmon) in a large bowl. Add the salmon fillets and coat with the yogurt mixture. Cover and refrigerate for at least 20-30 minutes.
2. Preheat a grill pan to a medium-high heat. Lightly grease the grill pan.
3. Remove the salmon from the yogurt mixture, ensuring the salmon is not covered in excess. Reserve the yogurt mixture in the bowl. Place the salmon fillets on the grill pan. Cook for about 10 minutes, turning after 5 minutes.
4. Arrange the salmon fillets on a serving plate and serve with a topping of the extra yogurt mixture.

CRISPY BAKED COD

A delicious alternative to fried fish that gets its great crunch from toasted breadcrumbs. Serve with baked potatoes or sweet potatoes.

SERVINGS 2
PREP TIME 10 MINS
COOK TIME 15 MINS

2 (6-ounce) pieces Cod Fillets
½ cup Gluten Free Breadcrumbs
1 tablespoon Fresh Parsley, finely chopped
1 tablespoon Extra Virgin Olive Oil
½ teaspoon Dried Thyme or Rosemary
½ teaspoon Salt

Directions

1. Preheat the oven to 425°F (220 degrees C). Place breadcrumbs in a baking sheet and bake, stirring once or twice, until lightly browned, about 5 minutes.
2. Transfer breadcrumbs to a medium bowl. Add parsley, oregano, oil and salt, and toss to combine.
3. Brush a baking sheet with oil. Press the breadcrumb mixture over both sides of cod pieces and arrange in the baking sheet. Press any remaining mixture over top of cod. Bake for about 12 minutes until fish flakes easily when pierced with a fork.

HERBED GRILLED TUNA STEAKS

These quick-and-easy grilled tuna steaks are rubbed with a simple mixture of herbs, salt, and olive oil prior to grilling. Serve these tuna steaks with rice and grilled vegetables.

SERVINGS 2

PREP TIME 15 MINS

COOK TIME 10 MINS

2 (5 ounces) Fresh Tuna Steaks
3 tablespoons Extra Virgin Olive Oil
1 teaspoon Fresh Thyme, minced
1 teaspoon Fresh Cilantro, minced
Salt, to taste

Directions

1. Combine the thyme, cilantro, oil and salt in a large bowl. Add the fish steaks and coat with the oil mixture. Cover and refrigerate for about 20-30 minutes.
2. Preheat a grill pan to a medium-high heat. Lightly grease the grill pan. Remove the fish from the oil mixture and discard any excess oil mixture.
3. Place the tuna steaks on the grill pan and cook for about 8-10 minutes. Turn the steaks after 5 minutes. Serve and enjoy!

BAKED FISH WITH CARROTS

The soft and scaly cod is ideal for toasting and cooking on baking sheets with carrots. This is a very tasty way to prepare cod that could not be simpler.

SERVINGS
2

PREP TIME
10 MINS

COOK TIME
15 MINS

2 (4-ounces) Cod, Haddock or Flounder Fillets
2-3 small Carrots, peeled and shredded
1 teaspoon Dried Rosemary, crushed
2 teaspoons Extra Virgin Olive Oil
Salt, to taste

Directions

1. Preheat the oven to 450°F (230 degrees C). Lightly grease two pieces of unfolded parchment papers.
2. Place one fish fillet over 1 piece of the parchment paper. Place half of the shredded carrots over the fish fillet. Sprinkle with rosemary and salt. Drizzle with the oil. Fold the parchment paper by sealing its edges with a narrow folder. Repeat the process with remaining fish fillet and piece of paper.
3. Place the parcels on a baking sheet, baking for about 15 minutes, or until done. Serve and enjoy!

CRAB CAKES

This tasty homemade crab cakes make the perfect summer dish for the whole family. The sweet, clean flavor of crab shines in this recipe for classic crab cakes.

SERVINGS
8

PREP TIME
15 MINS

COOK TIME
15 MINS

2 Eggs, beaten
1 pound Crabmeat, cooked
1 cup Cauliflower Florets, steamed well
3 tablespoons Coconut Flour
3 tablespoons Non-Dairy Plain Yogurt
2 tablespoons Fresh Parsley, chopped
½ teaspoon Ground Oregano
2 tablespoons Coconut Oil
½ teaspoon Salt

Directions

1. Place the steamed cauliflower in a medium bowl and gently break up into small pieces. Then, mash part of the cauliflower and leave some pieces intact for the crack cake's texture.
2. Add the crab meat and parsley into the bowl. Gently fold the mixture together until just combined, being careful not to break up the crab meat.

3. Whisk together the eggs, yogurt, oregano and salt in a small bowl. Pour over the crab meat mixture and gently fold.
4. Then, sift the coconut flour over the crab mixture and gently fold the mixture until everything is uniform. Cover and refrigerate for about 20-30 minutes. This helps them set.
5. Preheat oven to 350°F (175 degrees C).
6. Remove crab mixture from fridge and form into patties.
7. In a large skillet over medium-high heat, grease pan with oil and heat until shimmering. Add the crab cakes, being careful to not overcrowd the pan. Cook until golden brown, 3 to 5 minutes per side.
8. Place crab cakes on a baking sheet and transfer to the preheated oven. Bake for about 12 to 15 minutes.

GRILLED CHICKEN WITH KALE

This grilled chicken recipe not only comes with a combination of refreshing ingredients that will satisfy your taste buds, but also provides you with a wide variety of nutrients.

SERVINGS
2

PREP TIME
10 MINS

COOK TIME
25 MINS

1 large Chicken Breast, boneless skinless
¼ pound small Red Potatoes, cut into ½-inch pieces
½ large Bunch Kale, stems removed and leaves torn
2 tablespoons Extra Virgin Olive Oil
1 teaspoon Ground Oregano
Salt, as required

Directions

1. Preheat the oven to 425°F (220 degrees C). Toss the potatoes with ½ tablespoon olive oil on a rimmed baking sheet. Then, spread them in a single layer and roast for about 5 minutes.
2. In a large bowl, toss the kale with ½ tablespoon olive oil and ¼ teaspoon salt. Add to the baking sheet along the potatoes and toss. Roast for about 15 to 20 minutes until the potatoes are tender and the kale is crisp, stirring once.
3. Preheat a grill or grill pan to medium heat and lightly

grease with oil. Slice the chicken breast in half horizontally to make 4 pieces. Coat evenly with ½ tablespoon olive oil and season with oregano and salt. Cook the chicken for about 3-4 minutes until well marked and cooked through. Transfer to a plate.

4. In a large bowl, toss the potatoes, kale, the remaining ½ tablespoon olive oil and salt. Divide the pieces of chicken among plates and top with any collected juices. Serve with the kale salad and enjoy!

VEGETABLE TURKEY STEW

This turkey stew recipe is so cozy and delicious. It's super healthy and loaded with lean turkey and some vegetables, but it's also hearty enough to keep you full and satisfied.

SERVINGS: 2
PREP TIME: 15 MINS
COOK TIME: 20 MINS

½ pound Lean Ground Turkey
½ cup Vegetable Broth (see page 228)
2 Carrots, peeled and sliced into 1-inch pieces
¼ teaspoon Freshly Ground Coriander
½ teaspoon Freshly Ground Cumin
1 teaspoon Extra Virgin Olive Oil
1 Celery Stalk, minced
Salt, to taste

Directions

1. Heat the oil on a medium heat in a medium saucepan. Add the celery and sauté for 4 minutes. Add the cumin and coriander, and sauté for one more minute.
2. Add the turkey and cook, stirring frequently, for about 5 to 7 minutes. Add the remaining ingredients and increase the heat to high. Bring to the boil.
3. Once boiling, cover and simmer for about 8 to 10 minutes.
4. Serve warm and enjoy!

BAKED FISH WITH THYME CRUSTED

For a quick and light lunch or dinner nothing better than a healthy, protein packed fish baked with olive oil and thyme. Serve with rice or grilled vegetables.

SERVINGS
2

PREP TIME
10 MINS

COOK TIME
12 MINS

2 (4-ounces) Flounder, Haddock or Cod Fillets
1 tablespoon Dried Thyme, crushed
1 teaspoon Extra Virgin Olive Oil
Salt, to taste

Directions

1. Combine the oil and salt in a large mixing bowl. Add the fish fillets and coat with the oil mixture. Cover and refrigerate for about 20-30 minutes.
2. Preheat the oven to 450°F (230 degrees C). Line a baking sheet with a sheet of lightly greased foil.
3. Place dried thyme leaves in a shallow dish. Remove the fish from the oil mixture and coat with the dried thyme leaves.
4. Place the fish fillets on the prepared baking sheet and bake for about 12-15 minutes. Serve and enjoy!

GRILLED PRAWN SKEWERS

These delicious yogurt marinated skewers are perfect for a family barbecue weekend. Serve with your favorite side dish.

SERVINGS	PREP TIME	COOK TIME
2	15 MINS	6 MINS

2 Zucchinis, cut into chunks
½ cup Non-Dairy Plain Yogurt
6-8 Button Mushrooms, halved
¾ pound Tiger Prawns, shelled and halved lengthwise
½ teaspoon Freshly Ground Cumin
½ teaspoon Fresh Ginger, minced
1 tablespoon Fresh Basil, minced
Salt, to taste

Directions

1. In a medium shallow dish, combine the yogurt, cumin, ginger, basil and salt to make the marinade.
2. Thread the prawns, zucchini and mushrooms onto wooden skewers. Place the skewers in the dish and coat with the marinade. Cover and refrigerate to marinade for about 20-30 minutes.
3. Preheat the grill or grill pan over medium-high heat and lightly grease it. Remove the prawn skewers from the marinade.
4. Place the skewers on the grill and cook on both sides until prawns are cooked through (2-3 minutes on each side).

TILAPIA WITH SAUTÉED KALE

The combination of tilapia and kale makes this recipe a very nutritious one that provides a great variety of nutrients. Serve with baked potatoes or your favorite side dish.

SERVINGS: 2
PREP TIME: 10 MINS
COOK TIME: 10 MINS

2 (4-pound) Tilapia Fillets
1 teaspoon Fresh Rosemary, minced
3 tablespoons Extra Virgin Olive Oil
¾ pound Fresh Kale, trimmed and torn
Salt, to taste

Directions

1. Combine together 2 tablespoons of olive oil, rosemary and salt in a large mixing bowl. Add the tilapia fillets and coat with the oil mixture. Cover and refrigerate for about 20-30 minutes.
2. Preheat the grill or a grill pan over medium-high heat and lightly grease it. Remove the tilapia fillets from the oil mixture and discard any excess marinade. Place the tilapia fillets on the grill and cook for about 8-10 minutes, turning them after 5 minutes.
3. Heat the remaining oil on a medium heat in a skillet. Add the kale and sprinkle with a little of salt. Sauté for about 4-5 minutes. Remove from the heat.
4. Serve the grilled tilapia over the bed of sautéed kale.

BROILED SHRIMP

An easy recipe for very flavorful broiled shrimp with dried rosemary and olive oil seasoning. Serve with salad or your favorite side dish.

SERVINGS
2

PREP TIME
10 MINS

COOK TIME
5 MINS

1 teaspoon Extra Virgin Olive Oil
¾ pound large Shrimps, shelled and deveined
½ teaspoon Dried Rosemary, crushed
Salt, to taste

Directions

1. Turn on the broiler and put the rack close to the heat. Line a baking sheet with foil.
2. Place the shrimp on the prepared baking sheet in a single layer. Drizzle with the oil and sprinkle the rosemary and salt over the shrimp.
3. Broil for about 3-5 minutes. Then, remove from the heat and serve warm. Enjoy!

MAPLE-GLAZED SCALLOPS

A simple-to-make scallop dish that is dressed up with a super flavorful sweet and salty glaze.

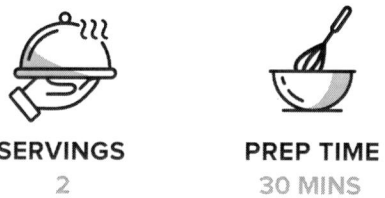

SERVINGS
2

PREP TIME
30 MINS

COOK TIME
10 MINS

8 Sea Scallops, tendons removed
1 teaspoon Miso Paste
¼ cup Maple Syrup
¼ teaspoon Ground Ginger (optional)
1 tablespoon Olive or Coconut Oil
½ teaspoon Salt

Directions

4. In a small mixing bowl, whisk together the maple syrup, miso, salt and ginger (if using). Add the scallops; toss to coat. Cover and refrigerate for 20 minutes.
5. In a large nonstick skillet, heat the oil over medium-high heat.
6. Add the scallops and cook until scallops are opaque, about 3-4 minutes on each side, basting occasionally with remaining marinade.
7. Serve and enjoy!

GRILLED CHICKEN WITH SPINACH

This grilled chicken and spinach recipe is a healthy option for lunch. It's low fat and rich in vitamins and proteins.

SERVINGS	PREP TIME	COOK TIME
2	12 MINS	20 MINS

3 cups Fresh Spinach, trimmed
2 (4-ounce) sliced boneless, skinless Chicken Breasts
1 tablespoon Extra Virgin Olive Oil
½ teaspoon Ground Oregano
1 teaspoon Dried Thyme
Salt, to taste

Directions

1. Preheat the grill or a grill pan over medium heat and lightly grease it.
2. Coat the chicken with half of the olive oil and sprinkle with thyme, oregano and salt. Cook the chicken for about 5 minutes on each side. Set aside the chicken and cover with foil to keep it warm.
3. Increase the heat to medium-high. Place greased foil paper on a smooth surface, and place the spinach in the center of the foil. Drizzle with the remaining olive oil and sprinkle with a little of salt. Fold the foil to seal it. Cook the spinach for about 8-10 minutes.
4. Place the spinach on a serving plate and place the chicken on top. Serve and enjoy!

TURKEY WITH KALE

This turkey and kale recipe is incredibly delicious, comforting and perfect for the busy weeknights. It's ready in less than 20 minutes.

SERVINGS
2

PREP TIME
15 MINS

COOK TIME
16 MINS

2 cups Kale
½ pound Lean Ground Turkey
1 teaspoon Extra Virgin Olive Oil
½ cup Vegetable Broth (see page 228)
¼ teaspoon Ground Cumin
1 Celery Stalk, minced
Salt, to taste

Directions

1. In a medium skillet, heat the oil over medium heat. Add the celery and sauté for about 4 minutes.
2. Add the turkey and cook, stirring frequently, for about 5-7 minutes. Add the kale, broth and cumin, and reduce the heat to low. Cook for further 6-8 minutes.
3. Season with salt and serve.

CHICKEN & RED LENTILS STEW

This chicken and lentil stew is the perfect midweek meal to warm you up in on a cold winter night.

SERVINGS
2

PREP TIME
15 MINS

COOK TIME
40 MINS

½ cup Red Lentils
½ pound Lean Ground Chicken
2 cups Chicken Broth (see page 226)
¼ teaspoon Freshly Ground Coriander
1 teaspoon Freshly Ground Cumin
½ tablespoon Dried Thyme
1½ tablespoons Extra Virgin Olive Oil
1 Celery Stalk, chopped finely
Salt, to taste

Directions

1. In a medium saucepan, heat the oil over medium heat. Add the celery and sauté for about 4 minutes. Then, add the cumin and coriander, and sauté for one more minute.
2. Add the chicken and cook, stirring frequently, for about 6-8 minutes. Add the remaining ingredients and bring to a boil. Reduce to a simmer and cook covered for about 30 minutes, stirring occasionally.
3. Serve warm and enjoy!

VEGGIE LOADED MEATLOAF

This is a filling and flavorful low-calorie meatloaf that is made healthier with the addition of veggies. Serve with mashed potatoes or your favorite side dish.

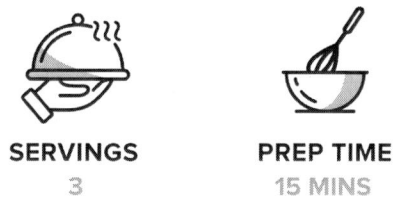

SERVINGS
3

PREP TIME
15 MINS

COOK TIME
1 HOUR

1 Egg, beaten
½ pound Lean Ground Turkey
½ pound Lean Ground Chicken
½ medium Yellow Squash, halved lengthwise
1 ½ tablespoons Mixed Dried Herbs (Oregano, Rosemary, Basil)
½ medium Zucchini, halved lengthwise
Salt, to taste

Directions

1. Preheat the oven to 350°F (175 degrees C). Lightly grease a loaf pan and set aside.
2. Combine the chicken, turkey, egg, herbs and salt in a large mixing bowl.
3. Place half of the meat mixture into the prepared pan. Then, press down from the center to make a shallow place. Sprinkle the squash and zucchini with the salt and place them in the center of the loaf pan, and gently press down. Top with the remaining meat mixture.
4. Cover and bake for about 45-55 minutes. Then, uncover the loaf pan and increase the temperature to 400°F. Bake for about 8-10 minutes.

BAKED SALMON WITH AVOCADO

This recipe combines two high-fat foods such as avocado and salmon that provides omega-3 fatty acids.

SERVINGS	PREP TIME	COOK TIME
2	20 MINS	15 MINS

½ Avocado
2 Salmon Fillets
¼ cup Almond Butter
1 teaspoon Honey or Maple Syrup
2 tablespoons Gluten Free Breadcrumbs
2 tablespoons Pecans, finely chopped
2 teaspoons Fresh Parsley, chopped
Salt to taste

Directions

1. Preheat oven to 400°F (205 degrees C).
2. Whisk together the butter and honey in a small bowl. Set aside. In another small bowl, mix the breadcrumbs, pecans, and parsley.
3. Brush each salmon fillet with the honey mixture. Then, sprinkle each salmon fillet with the breadcrumbs mixture.
4. Mash the avocado and season with salt. Set aside.
5. Bake the salmon in the preheated oven for about 12-15 minutes.
6. Serve with the avocado mixture and enjoy!

BAKED TURKEY MEATBALLS

These baked turkey meatballs are really popular with kids and adults alike. Serve them on skewers, with your favorite side dish, rolled in flat bread or just eat them straight from the pan.

SERVINGS
3

PREP TIME
10 MINS

COOK TIME
20 MINS

1 Egg, beaten
1-pound Lean Ground Turkey
½ cup Gluten Free Breadcrumbs
1 teaspoon Ground Cumin
¼ cup Leek, finely chopped
¼ cup Fresh Parsley, chopped
½ teaspoon Ground Oregano
½ teaspoon Salt

Directions

1. In a large bowl, combine all the ingredients and shape the mixture into 1½-inch meatballs.
2. Preheat the oven to 375°F. Lightly grease a baking sheet with nonstick spray oil. Set aside.
3. Place the meatballs in the prepared baking sheet and bake them for about 15-20 minutes or until the meatballs are cooked. Serve and enjoy!

CREAMY CHICKEN & BROCCOLI CASSEROLE

This healthy chicken broccoli casserole is a delicious comforting classic. It's so easy to make, packed with protein and loaded with broccoli.

SERVINGS
4

PREP TIME
15 MINS

COOK TIME
1 HOUR 15 MINS

1 large Egg
½ pound Mushrooms, sliced
½ head Broccoli, cut into thin slices
¾ head Cauliflower, cut into thin slices
2 (4-ounce) Chicken Breasts, boneless skinless
1 tablespoon Coconut Oil
½ cup Chicken Broth (see page 226)
½ cup Almonds, sliced
⅛ teaspoon Ground Oregano
1 cup Coconut Milk
⅛ teaspoon Salt

Directions

1. Heat the coconut oil in a non-stick skillet over medium-high heat.
2. Season chicken breasts with salt and sauté for about 10 minutes until fully cooked. Chop into bite-size pieces.
3. Preheat the oven to 350°F (175 degrees C).

4. Layer the cauliflower, broccoli, mushrooms, and cooked chicken in a baking dish, seasoning with salt between each layer.
5. In a medium bowl, whisk the egg with the coconut milk and chicken broth until well combined. Pour over the baking dish. Cover with foil and bake for about 30 minutes.
6. Remove from oven, uncover and sprinkle with sliced almonds. Bake uncovered for about 5 to 10 minutes until almonds are lightly toasted and casserole is bubbly.
7. Let sit for about 5 to 10 minutes before serving. Enjoy!

ZUCCHINI SHRIMP SCAMPI

This easy zucchini shrimp scampi recipe is just like the traditional recipe except the pasta has been replaced with spiralized zucchini.

SERVINGS: 2
PREP TIME: 10 MINS
COOK TIME: 15 MINS

4 medium Zucchinis
1 tablespoon Extra Virgin Olive Oil
1-pound medium Shrimp, peeled and deveined
1 teaspoon Dried Thyme
¼ cup Chicken Broth (see page 226)
Parsley, for garnish
1 teaspoon Salt

Directions

1. Make zucchini noodles using a spiralizer or julienne peeler.
2. In a large nonstick skillet, heat the oil over medium-high heat.
3. Add the shrimp in and season with the thyme and salt. Sauté the shrimp for about 2 to 3 minutes until they begin to turn pink.
4. Pour in the chicken broth and let the liquid come to a simmer.
5. Add the zucchini noodles and stir until well combined and the shrimp are fully cooked.
6. Sprinkle with chopped fresh parsley. Serve and enjoy!

COCONUT CHICKEN WITH SPINACH

A tasty and easy to prepare recipe that uses a handful of simple, nutritious ingredients. Coconut-based ingredients are rich in healthy fats, which is ideal if you don't want to lose weight.

SERVINGS 2
PREP TIME 10 MINS
COOK TIME 15 MINS

1 large Chicken Breast
3 cups Baby Spinach
½ cup canned Coconut Milk
3 tablespoons Coconut Oil
A handful of Almonds
Pinch of Ground Oregano
Salt, to taste

Directions

1. In a medium saucepan, add the spinach and coconut milk. Cook covered on a simmer.
2. Add the almonds in a food processor and pulse until chopped. Then lightly brown them in a pan with coconut oil. Set aside.
3. Cut the chicken breast into cubes, add it to the pan and leave until thoroughly cooked.
4. Add the chicken to the pot with the spinach and coconut milk. Stir and cover for 2 more minutes.
5. Serve garnished with toasted almonds, and salt.

BAKED PORTOBELLO & SALMON

Thick and meaty portobello mushrooms replace bread to make this delicious baked salmon recipe. Serve with a side of steamed vegetables.

SERVINGS 2　　**PREP TIME** 15 MINS　　**COOK TIME** 20 MINS

1 Egg, lightly beaten
1 can (6 oz) Salmon, drained
½ cup Gluten Free Breadcrumbs
2 medium Portobello Mushrooms
2 teaspoons Fresh Dill, chopped (optional)
1 tablespoon Extra Virgin Olive Oil
2 tablespoons Capers, rinsed
¼ teaspoon Ground Cumin
¼ teaspoon Ground Oregano
½ medium Avocado, sliced
½ teaspoon Salt

Directions

1. Preheat oven to 450°F (230 degrees C).
2. Clean mushrooms, remove stems, and carefully scrape gills away using a spoon.
3. Combine the salmon, breadcrumbs, egg, cumin, oregano,

dill (if using) and capers in a medium bowl. Then, stuff into portobello caps.
4. Grease a baking sheet with the olive oil and place the caps. Bake for about 15-20 minutes until tops are browned and portobello cap has softened.
5. Top with sliced avocado and serve warm. Enjoy!

SHRIMP AVOCADO OMELETTE

This simple, elegant omelet is the perfect centerpiece for an extra special meal. Loaded with shrimp and avocado, this dish will surely satisfy you.

SERVINGS
2

PREP TIME
15 MINS

COOK TIME
30 MINS

4 large Eggs, beaten
½ medium Avocado, diced
¼ pound Shrimp, peeled and deveined
1 tablespoon Fresh Cilantro, chopped
⅛ teaspoon Ground Oregano
1 teaspoon Coconut Oil
¼ teaspoon Salt

Directions

1. In a nonstick skillet, add the shrimp and cook over medium heat until pink. Chop and set aside.
2. In a small bowl, toss together avocado and cilantro. Season with oregano and salt to taste. Set aside.
3. Beat eggs in a separate bowl.
4. Heat the coconut oil in a nonstick skillet over medium-high heat.
5. Pour half of the eggs into the hot skillet. As the eggs are

cooked, lift the edges and slightly tilt the pan to cover the sides and allow the raw part to flow underneath.
6. Once eggs are cooked, add shrimp pieces onto one half of the egg and fold omelette in half and cook for a further minute.
7. Top with avocado mixture. Repeat for second omelet.

ALMOND CRUSTED TILAPIA

This almond crusted tilapia is a simple and delicious way to add seafood to your weekly dinner menu. It's light, healthy, and super easy.

SERVINGS: 2
PREP TIME: 15 MINS
COOK TIME: 15 MINS

1 Egg, beaten
2 (6-ounce) Tilapia Fillets
½ cup Almond Flour
1 teaspoon Dried Rosemary or Thyme, minced
3 tablespoons Dairy-free Parmesan cheese (optional)
1 tablespoon Coconut Oil
¼ teaspoon Salt

Directions

1. In a medium mixing bowl, combine almond flour, rosemary, salt and dairy-free parmesan (if using).
2. Dip each fillet in egg and then in almond flour mixture. Make sure each fillet is completely coated.
3. Heat the oil in a medium skillet over medium-high heat. Add the tilapia fillets and cook for about 2-3 minutes per side, or until fish flakes easily with a fork.
4. Remove fillets to a serving plate. Serve and enjoy!

CHICKEN ZUCCHINI MEATBALLS

These baked chicken zucchini meatballs are great added to your favorite dishes and deliver extra nutrition thanks to the addition of zucchini.

SERVINGS 4
PREP TIME 20 MINS
COOK TIME 25 MINS

1-pound Lean Ground Chicken
2 medium Zucchinis, grated and water squeezed out
4 tablespoons Fresh Cilantro, minced
½ teaspoon Ground Cumin
½ teaspoon Ground Oregano
Olive Oil Cooking Spray, as required
½ teaspoon Salt

Directions

1. Preheat oven to 400°F (205 degrees C). Grease a baking sheet with nonstick cooking spray. Set aside.
2. In a medium bowl, combine ground chicken, zucchini, cilantro, oregano, cumin and salt.
3. Roll chicken mixture into about 1 - 1½ inch meatballs and place on the greased baking sheet.
4. Bake for about 20-25 minutes, or until cooked through. Place under the broiler for an additional 2-3 minutes or until browned on top (watch them carefully so they don't burn).

COCONUT FISH STICKS

These healthy fish sticks are a great alternative to the deep fried, processed flour coated favorite. Serve with your favorite side dish.

SERVINGS	PREP TIME	COOK TIME
2	10 MINS	20 MINS

¾ pounds Cod or Tilapia Fillets
1 ½ cups Coconut Flakes
2 tablespoons Coconut Aminos or Braggs Liquid Aminos
½ cup Non-Dairy Plain Yogurt
1 Egg

Directions

1. Preheat oven to 400°F (205 degrees C). Put the oven rack in the top or bottom third of the oven. Line a baking sheet and lightly grease it with non-stick cooking spray.
2. Cut the fish filets in half lengthwise down the center line. Half again lengthwise then cut in half crosswise.
3. In a shallow dish, beat the egg with 1 tablespoon coconut aminos. Place the coconut flakes on a separate plate.
4. Dip the strips of fish into the egg mixture, then into the coconut, pressing to adhere. Place on the prepared baking sheet and spray lightly with cooking spray. Bake for about 15 to 20 minutes until lightly golden brown.
5. Whisk the remaining coconut aminos with the yogurt. Serve the fish sticks with the sauce.

TURKEY QUINOA MEATLOAF

The secret ingredient in this flavorful turkey meatloaf is quinoa. Quinoa is nuttier than breadcrumbs and improves the texture of the meatloaf.

SERVINGS
4

PREP TIME
10 MINS

COOK TIME
1 HOUR

2 Eggs, beaten
¼ cup Uncooked Quinoa
1 pound Lean Ground Turkey
½ teaspoon Ground Cumin
1 teaspoon Extra Virgin Olive Oil
1 teaspoon Thyme, minced
1 teaspoon Rosemary, minced
¼ teaspoon Ground Oregano
1 teaspoon Salt

Directions

1. Rinse the quinoa for two or three minutes in a fine metal strainer. (Skip this step if you using pre-rinsed quinoa).
2. Add one part quinoa to about two parts water. Bring to a boil and then reduce heat to low. Cook covered for about 15-20 minutes until the quinoa is tender, and the water has been absorbed. Set aside to cool.
3. Preheat oven to 350 degrees F (175 degrees C).
4. Combine cooked quinoa and all other ingredients in a large mixing bowl. Then, grease a loaf pan with olive oil and add the mixture. Bake for 1 hour. Serve and enjoy!

ZUCCHINI WRAPPED FISH

This zucchini wrapped fish recipe is one of those great dishes that looks fancy but is actually quite simple.

SERVINGS 2

PREP TIME 10 MINS

COOK TIME 8 MINS

1 (6-inch long) Zucchini, trimmed

2 (6-ounce) Halibut Fillets, skinned

3 tablespoons Extra-Virgin Olive Oil, divided

1 teaspoon Dried Thyme

8 Fresh Basil Leaves

Salt, to taste

Directions

1. Slice the zucchini into thin pieces lengthwise with a peeler or mandoline.
2. Season the fish fillets with ½ tsp. dried thyme, 1 tablespoon olive oil and salt.
3. Arrange about 5 slices of zucchini on a work surface, side by side, overlapping each slice by half. Brush zucchini with oil, then lightly season with salt and dried thyme. Lay 2 basil leaves across center of each group of zucchini slices.
4. Arrange fish crosswise on zucchini, covering basil leaves. Top each piece of fish with 2 basil leaves, then wrap zucchini around fish, overlapping ends.

5. Put 1 tablespoon oil in a nonstick skillet and swirl to coat bottom, then arrange fish, seam sides down, in oil. Lightly brush tops of zucchini and fish with oil.
6. Cover skillet and cook fish over medium heat, without turning, until barely cooked through, 7 to 10 minutes, depending on thickness of fillets.
7. Transfer fish to plates, then add the remaining oil and season with salt.

TURKEY BROCCOLI & RICE CASSEROLE

This is a simple, healthy turkey and rice casserole. Turn your leftover cooked turkey into a tasty new skillet dish.

SERVINGS
8

PREP TIME
15 MINS

COOK TIME
45 MINS

¾ cup Cashews
3 cups Cooked White Rice
2 cups Cooked Shredded Turkey
3 cups Broccoli, chopped into small florets
4 cups Chicken Broth, divided (see page 226)
2 tablespoons Gluten Free Flour
4-ounce Cremini Mushrooms, finely chopped
2 tablespoon Fresh Parsley, chopped
1-2 teaspoons Coconut Aminos
2 tablespoons Coconut Oil
Salt, to taste

Directions

1. Preheat the oven to 375°F (190 degrees C). Pour 1 cup of boiling water over the cashews and let sit for about 25-30 minutes while you prepare the rest of the ingredients.
2. Heat the oil over medium heat in a large dutch oven until shimmering. Add the mushrooms, parsley, and a pinch

of salt. Cook for about 7 to 10 minutes until softened. Sprinkle the flour over the mushroom mixture and cook for about 2-3 minutes.

3. Slowly pour in 3 cups of the chicken broth while whisking continuously. Bring to a simmer and cook for about 5 minutes, until thickened.
4. Drain and rinse the cashews. Place them in a high-speed blender with ½ cup of chicken broth and blend until smooth. Mix the cashews along with the coconut aminos.
5. Stir the turkey, white rice and broccoli into the cashews mix. Taste and season with additional salt if needed. Add up to ½ cup additional chicken broth if the mixture looks too thick. Pour into a greased 3-quart casserole dish. Bake for about 25-30 minutes until bubbly and golden on top.
6. Serve and enjoy!

CHAPTER 8

SALAD & SOUP RECIPES

APPLE WALNUT KALE SALAD

This walnut apple kale salad that is nothing but refreshing, nutrient dense and full of vitamins, minerals and fiber.

SERVINGS 2
PREP TIME 12 MINS
COOK TIME 8 MINS

1 Red Apple, peeled, cored and chopped
3 cups Fresh Kale, ribs removed and chopped
½ tablespoon Extra Virgin Olive Oil
½ tablespoon Maple Syrup
1 Celery Stalk, chopped
⅓ cup Walnut halves
Salt, to taste

Directions

1. Grease a nonstick skillet with oil over medium heat. Add the celery and kale. Cook, stirring occasionally, until kale wilted and celery have softened, 6-8 minutes. Remove from the heat and set aside.
2. In a large bowl, add the apple, kale, celery and walnuts.
3. In a separate bowl, add remaining ingredients and mix everything until well combined
4. Pour maple syrup and toss to coat well. Serve and enjoy!

CARROT WALDORF SALAD

Tasty combo of apple chunks, chewy raisins, crunchy walnuts and sweet carrots make this salad a big hit.

SERVINGS 2 | **PREP TIME** 10 MINS | **COOK TIME** 5 MINS

1 cup Red Apple, chopped
2 tablespoons Walnuts, chopped
2 tablespoons Raisins
1 cup Carrots, peeled and shredded
¼ cup Non-Dairy Plain Yogurt
¼-inch of Fresh Ginger, peeled and chopped
1 tablespoon Extra Virgin Olive Oil
1 tablespoon Maple Syrup
¼ cup Carrot Juice
Pinch of Salt

Directions

1. In a large nonstick skillet, heat the oil over medium-high heat. Add carrots and cook, stirring continuously, until slightly softened, about 3-4 minutes.
2. In a large mixing bowl, add the apple, shredded carrots, walnuts and raisins. Stir to combine.
3. Whisk together the yogurt, carrot juice, maple syrup, ginger and salt in a separate bowl.
4. Pour yogurt mixture over carrot mixture and toss. Cover, and chill at least 1 hour before serving.

AVOCADO MANGO BROCCOLI SALAD

A delicious recipe for those days when you are super busy and want a healthy salad in 15 minutes or less.

SERVINGS: 2
PREP TIME: 15 MINS
COOK TIME: N/A

1 ripe Mangoes, cubed
1 ripe Avocados, cubed
1 cup Cooked Broccoli, cut into bite size pieces
¼ cup Slivered Almonds, toasted
1 tablespoon Extra-Virgin Olive Oil
Salt, to taste

Directions

1. In a large mixing bowl, mix together all ingredients.
2. Drizzle with olive oil. Sprinkle with salt.
3. Gently, toss to coat well. Serve and enjoy!

FRESH FRUIT SALAD

This refreshing fruit salad not only tastes good and is comforting, but also contains a great variety of fruits rich in antioxidants and with anti-inflammatory properties.

SERVINGS
2

PREP TIME
15 MINS

COOK TIME
N/A

1 cup Banana, chopped
½ cup Fresh Papaya, cubed
1 cup Honeydew Melon, cubed
1 cup Watermelon, peeled, seeded and cubed
¼ cup Fresh Blueberries
1 tablespoon Maple Syrup
Pinch of Salt

Directions

1. In a large mixing bowl, mix together fruits.
2. In a separate bowl, beat together maple syrup and salt.
3. Pour maple syrup dressing over salad and toss to coat well.
4. Cover and refrigerate to chill completely before serving.

MOROCCAN CARROT & SPINACH SALAD

This sweet Moroccan carrot salad is loaded with delicious good-for-you ingredients. Carrots are rich in vitamin A, which keep your eyes healthy.

SERVINGS
4

PREP TIME
15 MINS

COOK TIME
10 MINS

2 ½ cups Carrots, sliced on the bias
2 ½ tablespoons Extra Virgin Olive Oil
1 ½ cups Fresh Baby Spinach or Kale
¼-inch of Fresh Ginger, peeled and chopped
¼ teaspoon Ground Cumin
¼ cup Carrot Juice
2 tablespoon Maple Syrup
¾ teaspoon Salt

Directions

1. In a large sauté pan heat 1 tablespoon olive oil. Add the carrots, 1 tablespoon maple syrup, and ½ teaspoon salt. Cook carrots until they just start softening. Turn off heat and allow to sit for a few minutes.
2. In another sauté pan heat ½ tablespoon olive oil. Add the spinach and cook briefly – just until wilted. Remove from the pan and rough chop.
3. In a large bowl add the drained cooked carrots and spinach. Mix together carrot juice, ginger, cumin, remaining salt, olive oil and maple syrup, and pour over salad. Serve warm or at room temp.

APPLE & CARROT SALAD

Shredded carrot salad with apple and walnuts has a touch of maple syrup to make for a sweet, fresh and healthy side dish.

SERVINGS
3

PREP TIME
15 MINS

COOK TIME
5 MINS

½ cup Walnut Kernels
3 medium Carrots, cut into matchsticks
1 Apple, peeled, cut into matchsticks
2 tablespoons Extra Virgin Olive Oil
1 tablespoon Maple Syrup
¼ cup Sultanas
Salt, to taste

Directions:

1. Preheat oven to 355°F (180 degrees C). Place the walnuts and carrots on a baking sheet. Bake for about 5 minutes. Set aside.
2. Place the apple in a bowl. Add the walnuts, sultanas and carrots.
3. Combine oil and maple syrup in a small bowl. Season with salt. Drizzle over salad and toss to combine. Serve and enjoy!

QUINOA & KALE SALAD

A simple, healthy and satisfying quinoa salad with kale and sliced almonds.

SERVINGS
4

PREP TIME
15 MINS

COOK TIME
20 MINS

1 cup Quinoa, rinsed

3 cups Kale, stems removed and finely chopped

¼ cup toasted Almonds, sliced

½ medium Avocado, cubed

¼-inch Fresh Ginger, peeled and chopped

½ cup Carrot Juice

1 tablespoon Extra Virgin Olive Oil

1 tablespoon Maple Syrup

1 ½ cups Water

¼ teaspoon of Salt

Directions

4. In a medium saucepan, combine the quinoa and water. Bring the water to a boil, reduce the heat to low and cover. Cook until all of the water is absorbed, about 15-20 minutes. Fluff the quinoa with a fork.
5. Transfer the cooked quinoa into a bowl, and place in the refrigerator until it cools.

6. In a small bowl, whisk together the olive oil, carrot juice, ginger, maple syrup and salt. Cover and set this dressing aside.
7. To the cooked quinoa, add the kale, almonds, and avocado. Stir to combine.
8. Pour the dressing over the quinoa salad and stir to combine. Serve at room temperature or cold.

GINGER-SESAME VEGGIE SALAD

This is an excellent vegetarian Chinese-style stir-fry. It's perfect for lunch or dinner and ideal for serving with some white rice or cauliflower rice.

SERVINGS 2
PREP TIME 25 MINS
COOK TIME 10 MINS

1 large Carrots, julienned
2 cups Fresh Broccoli, cut into florets
½ cup Green Beans, cut into 2-inch pieces
1 cup Fresh Spinach
¼ cup Walnuts, chopped
¼ cup Coconut Aminos or Bragg Liquid Aminos
2 tablespoons Sesame Oil
½ tablespoon Arrowroot Flour or NON-GMO Cornstarch
1 tablespoon Fresh Gingerroot, grated

Directions

1. In a small bowl, mix together coconut aminos, sesame oil, arrowroot flour and ginger.
2. In a stockpot, place a steamer basket over 2 inches of water. Place carrots, green beans and broccoli in basket. Bring water to a boil. Reduce heat to a simmer and cook covered for about 5-7 minutes or just until vegetables are crisp-tender. Add spinach and cook covered for further 1-2 minutes or until spinach is wilted.
3. Transfer vegetables to a large mixing bowl. Add ginger mixture and toss to combine. Serve and enjoy!

AVOCADO EGG SALAD

A nutritious salad of avocado and egg that provides lots of healthy fats and high-quality proteins.

SERVINGS: 2
PREP TIME: 15 MINS
COOK TIME: N/A

2 Eggs
1 Avocado, peeled and pitted
1 tablespoon Non-Dairy Yogurt
A handful of Parsley
Salt, to taste

Directions

1. Place eggs in a saucepan and cover with water. Bring to a boil, remove from heat, and let eggs stand in hot water for 15 minutes.
2. Remove eggs from hot water, cool under cold running water, and peel. Chop eggs and transfer to a bowl.
3. Mash avocado in a separate bowl using a fork. Mix mashed avocado, parsley and yogurt into eggs until thoroughly combined. Season with salt to taste.
4. Serve and enjoy!

HERBED SUMMER SQUASH SALAD

This is a delicious way to prepare your squashes from the garden veggies. It has a very summery taste.

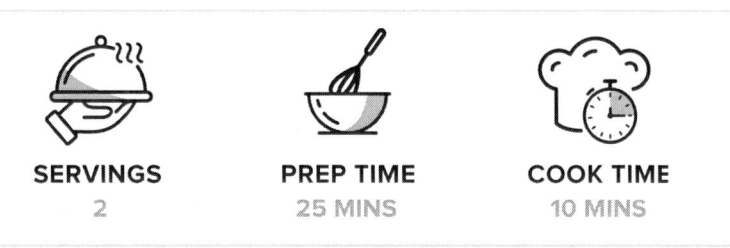

SERVINGS 2

PREP TIME 25 MINS

COOK TIME 10 MINS

¼ pound Zucchini, sliced thinly
¼ pound Summer Squash, sliced thinly
1 tablespoon Extra Virgin Olive Oil
1 teaspoon Fresh Thyme, minced
1 teaspoon Fresh Parsley, minced
1 teaspoon Fresh Basil, minced
Pinch of Salt

Directions

1. Coat a nonstick skillet with olive oil on medium-high heat. Add the summer squash and zucchini and salt to taste. Cook, stirring occasionally, until they are translucent, about 10 minutes.
2. In a small bowl, add remaining ingredients and mix until well combined
3. Pour dressing over salad and toss to coat well.
4. Cover and refrigerate for about 3-4 hours.

KALE & ZUCCHINI SOUP

This recipe for hearty kale and zucchini soup is a nice change from ordinary soups and stews and a real palate pleaser.

SERVINGS
2

PREP TIME
15 MINS

COOK TIME
25 MINS

¼ cup Celery, chopped
½ cup Zucchini, chopped
1 cup Fresh Kale, chopped
2 tablespoons Fresh Basil, chopped
2 cups Vegetable Broth (see page 228)
2 tablespoons Almonds, toasted and chopped
1 teaspoon Extra Virgin Olive Oil
Salt, to taste

Directions

1. In a medium stockpot, heat oil over medium heat. Add celery, zucchini and basil and sauté for 5-6 minutes. Add vegetable broth and bring to a boil. Reduce the heat to medium-low and then simmer for about 10 minutes.
2. Add kale and simmer for 5 minutes. Stir in almonds and remove from heat. Let it cool slightly. In a blender, add soup and puree in batches until smooth.
3. Add soup in the stockpot again and season with salt. Cook for about 3-4 minutes on medium-low-heat. Serve and enjoy!

CREAMY BROCCOLI SOUP

This creamy super-healthy broccoli soup does not require any cream or butter to get its creamy texture. Ideal to accompany with slices of crusty toast.

SERVINGS
2

PREP TIME
15 MINS

COOK TIME
4 MINS

2 cups Steamed Broccoli
⅓ cup Steamed Carrots, chopped
1 ½ cups Fresh Spinach, chopped
¼ cup canned Coconut Milk
1 cup Vegetable Broth (see page 228)
1 teaspoon Extra Virgin Olive Oil
¼ cup Fresh Basil Leaves
Salt, to taste

Directions

1. In a blender, add all ingredients (except olive oil) and pulse until smooth.
2. Transfer the mixture into a saucepan and heat completely for about 2-4 minutes.
3. Drizzle with olive oil and serve warm. Enjoy!

PUMPKIN & SWEET POTATO SOUP

This creamy sweet potato and pumpkin soup has a soft texture, making it a perfect dish for the fall months.

SERVINGS
2

PREP TIME
15 MINS

COOK TIME
30 MINS

2 small Sweet Potatoes, peeled and chopped
¼ pound Pumpkin, peeled, seeded and chopped
4 cups Vegetable Broth (see page 228)
1 teaspoon Extra-Virgin Olive Oil
½ cup Leek (white part only), chopped
1 tablespoon Fresh Basil, chopped
1 Celery Stalk, chopped
Salt, to taste

Directions

1. In a medium stockpot, heat oil over medium heat. Add celery and leek and sauté for 2 minutes. Add vegetable broth, pumpkin and sweet potato. Bring to a boil. Then, reduce the heat to low. Simmer for about 25-30 minutes.
2. Remove from heat and let it cool slightly. In a blender, add soup and puree in batches until smooth.
3. Return the soup into the stockpot and cook for about 2-3 minutes or until heated completely. Add salt as necessary and serve warm. Enjoy!

CHICKEN & KALE SOUP

This light and comforting soup is loaded with kale and chicken. It is healthy, full of nutrients and ideal for a light meal in the middle of the week.

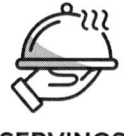

SERVINGS
2

PREP TIME
10 MINS

COOK TIME
35 MINS

1 Celery Stalk, chopped
½ cup leek (white part only), washed and finely chopped
1 Chicken Breast, sliced into thin strips
1 ½ cups Kale, ribs removed and chopped
2 small Carrots, peeled and chopped
3 cups Chicken Broth (see page 226)
1 tablespoon Fresh Basil, chopped
Salt, to taste

Directions

1. In a medium stockpot, add vegetable broth, chicken, leek, carrots, celery and basil. Bring to a boil. Reduce the heat to medium-low and cook for about 25-35 minutes.
2. Remove chicken from soup and cool slightly. Shred the chicken and return it in the stockpot again. Add kale and cook for about 4-5 minutes.
3. Season with salt and serve warm. Enjoy!

LENTIL SPINACH SOUP

A delicious vegetarian soup filled with spinach and red lentils. Ideal to accompany with slices of crusty toast.

SERVINGS: 2
PREP TIME: 15 MINS
COOK TIME: 25 MINS

½ cup Red Lentils, rinsed
1 medium Carrot, peeled and chopped
½ cup leek (white part only), washed and finely chopped
½ large Bunch Spinach, chopped roughly
3 cups Low-sodium Vegetable Broth (see page 228)
1 teaspoon Fresh Thyme, chopped
Salt, to taste

Directions

1. In a medium stockpot, add vegetable broth, lentils and vegetables and bring to a boil over medium-high heat.
2. Reduce the heat to medium-low. Cover and then simmer for about 15-20 minutes.
3. Stir in thyme and salt. Remove from heat and let it cool slightly. In a blender, add soup and puree in batches until smooth.
4. Return the soup into the stockpot and cook for about 2-3 minutes or until heated completely. Add salt as necessary and serve warm. Enjoy!

CHICKPEAS & CELERY SOUP

A comforting, hearty and healthy vegetable soup packed with chickpeas and celery stalks. So simple to make, too!

SERVINGS 2   **PREP TIME** 15 MINS   **COOK TIME** 15 MINS

2 Celery Stalks, chopped
2 cups Cooked Chickpeas
2 cups Low-sodium Chicken Broth (see page 226)
½ teaspoon Extra-Virgin Olive Oil
1 Sprig Fresh Rosemary
Pinch of Ground Cumin
Pinch of Salt

Directions

1. In a blender, add half of the chickpeas, cumin, rosemary, salt and some chicken broth and pulse according to your desired texture.
2. In a medium stockpot, add the chickpea mixture, celery, remaining chickpeas and chicken broth and cook for approximately 10-15 minutes or until desired consistency.
3. Drizzle with olive oil and serve warm.

MISO SOUP

Miso soup is a staple of Japanese cuisine. This recipe is a simple version of the classic vegetarian miso soup served in Japanese restaurants.

SERVINGS
3

PREP TIME
10 MINS

COOK TIME
5 MINS

3 cups Dashi or Low-sodim Vegetable Broth
¼ cup Dried Wakame
2 tablespoons White Miso Paste
6-ounce Soft or Firm Tofu, cut into ½-inch cubes
¼ cup Leek, thinly sliced

Directions

1. In a bowl, combine wakame with warm water to cover by 1-inch and let sit for about 15 minutes, or until reconstituted. Drain in a strainer.
2. In a small bowl, stir together miso and ½ cup dashi until smooth.
3. Heat remaining dashi or broth in a medium saucepan over medium-high heat until hot, then gently stir in tofu and wakame. Simmer for 1 minute and remove from heat.
4. Stir in miso mixture and leek and serve warm. Enjoy!

ROASTED WINTER SQUASH SOUP

The secret to the intense taste of this soup is to roast the squash in the oven until it is completely browned and caramelized.

SERVINGS
2

PREP TIME
20 MINS

COOK TIME
1 HOUR 30 MINS

½ Celery Stalk, chopped
1 Small Carrot, peeled and chopped
1 Small Butternut Squash, halved and seeded (about 2 cups)
⅓ leek (white part only), washed and sliced
2 cups Low-sodium Vegetable Broth (see page 228)
2 tablespoons Non-Dairy Plain Yogurt (optional)
Pinch of Ground Cumin
1 teaspoon Extra Virgin Olive Oil
Salt, to taste

Directions

1. Preheat the oven to 350°F (175 degrees C). Line a baking sheet with foil paper. Place winter squash halves on prepared baking sheet, cut side down. Roast for approximately 45-55 minutes. Discard the pulp and transfer into a bowl. Set aside.
2. In a medium stockpot, heat oil over medium-low heat. Stir in celery, leek and carrot. Cook covered, stirring

occasionally, for about 8-10 minutes. Add cumin and cook by stirring for 1 minute. Add broth and squash and bring to a boil. Reduce the heat to low. Cover and simmer for about 15-20 minutes. Remove from heat and let it slightly cool.
3. In a blender, add soup and puree in batches until smooth. Return the soup into the stockpot and cook for about 2-3 minutes or until heated completely. Season with salt.
4. Top with yogurt (if using) and serve warm with gluten-free toast. Enjoy!

CREAMY CARROT SOUP

This creamy carrot soup is a wonderful way to enjoy carrots rich in beta-carotene, especially during the cold autumn and winter months.

SERVINGS: 2
PREP TIME: 15 MINS
COOK TIME: 15 MINS

1 cup Carrots, diced
½ Celery Stalk, chopped finely
¼ teaspoon Ground Cumin
¼ teaspoon Ground Coriander
¼ teaspoon Dried Thyme, crushed
1 teaspoon Extra-Virgin Olive Oil
1 cup Low-sodium Vegetable Broth (see page 228)
2 tablespoons Fresh Parsley
Salt, to taste

Directions

1. In a medium stockpot, heat oil on medium heat. Add celery and sauté for about 2 to 3 minutes. Add seasonings and sauté for a further minute.
2. In a blender, add ¾ cup of carrots and some water and puree until smooth. Transfer the pureed carrots in stockpot. Add broth and bring to a boil.
3. Reduce the heat to medium-low, add remaining carrots and simmer for about 15 minutes. Stir in parsley and serve.

CREAMY SHRIMP & RICE SOUP

This creamy shrimp soup tastes rich without being as heavy as most cream soups. Perfect for those cold winter days.

SERVINGS
2

PREP TIME
30 MINS

COOK TIME
45 MINS

⅓ cup White Rice
½ cup Carrot, thinly sliced
½ pound Medium-sized Shrimp, peeled and deveined
½ small Leek, thinly sliced and well rinsed
1 teaspoon Dried or Fresh Dill weed, chopped
4 cups Fresh Spinach, coarsely chopped
2 ½ cups Low-sodium Chicken Broth (see page 226)
1 tablespoon Fresh Parsley, chopped
½ cup Non-Dairy Plain Yogurt
½ teaspoon Salt

Directions

1. In a large saucepan, bring the broth to a boil. Stir in the rice and salt. Reduce heat and simmer, covered, for about 12-14 minutes. Stir in parsley and carrot. Simmer, covered, 5 minutes more or until carrots are tender and rice is done.
2. Stir in yogurt and bring to a boil, then reduce heat and simmer, covered, for about 5 minutes. Stir in shrimp and leek. Simmer, covered, 3-4 minutes or until shrimp are opaque. Add spinach and cook stirring until wilted. Then stir in dill. Serve warm and enjoy!

CHAPTER 9

SIDE DISH & VEGAN RECIPES

BUTTERNUT SQUASH AND KALE

This sautéed butternut squash tossed with kale and fresh herbs is a great side dish for the holidays.

SERVINGS: 2
PREP TIME: 10 MINS
COOK TIME: 10 MINS

1 Bunch Kale, stems removed and leaves torn
½ Butternut Squash, peeled, seeded and cubed
1 ½ tablespoons Fresh Herbs (Rosemary, Thyme, Oregano)
2 tablespoons Extra Virgin Olive Oil
Pinch of Freshly Ground Cumin
½ teaspoon Salt

Directions

1. In a large nonstick skillet, heat 1 tablespoon olive oil over medium-high heat. Add squash and sprinkle with salt, cumin and herbs. Cook for several minutes, turning gently with a spatula, until squash is golden brown and tender. Remove to a plate and set aside.
2. In the same skillet, heat the remaining olive oil over medium-high heat and add in the kale. Toss it around and cook for about 3 to 4 minutes. Add in the cooked squash and toss together. Serve and enjoy!

SQUASHES & CHICKPEAS

This delicious combination of pumpkin and chickpeas is based on a traditional Moroccan recipe known as harira. It is a delicious protein-rich dish from chickpeas.

SERVINGS	PREP TIME	COOK TIME
2	15 MINS	20 MINS

1 ½ cups Cooked Chickpeas
2 cups Yellow Squash, cut into ½-inch slices
2 cups Butternut Squash, cut into ½-inch slices
2 cups Zucchini, cut into ½-inch slices
½ cup Low-sodium Vegetable Broth (see page 228)
2 teaspoons Extra-Virgin Olive Oil
½ teaspoon Ground Cumin
Salt, to taste

Directions

1. In a medium skillet, heat oil over medium heat. Add squashes and sauté for about 4-5 minutes.
2. Add remaining ingredients and bring to a boil. Reduce heat to low. Cover and simmer, stirring occasionally, for about 10 to 15 minutes. Serve warm and enjoy!

ROASTED BROCCOLI CHICKPEA QUINOA

A veggie bowl recipe for vegans loaded with roasted broccoli and chickpeas and fluffy quinoa in a maple dressing.

SERVINGS 2

PREP TIME 10 MINS

COOK TIME 30 MINS

¾ cup Uncooked Quinoa
1 cup canned Organic Chickpeas, drained and rinsed well
1 small Bunch Broccoli, cut into mini florets (about 3 cups)
½ cup Fresh Parsley, roughly chopped
1 ½ cups Water or Vegetable Broth
4 tablespoons Extra Virgin Olive Oil
1 tablespoon Maple Syrup
⅛ teaspoon Dried Dill (optional)
Pinch of Salt

Directions

1. Preheat oven to 400°F (205 degrees C). Line a baking sheet with parchment paper.
2. Transfer chickpeas and broccoli to the prepared baking sheet and drizzle with 1 tablespoon olive oil and sprinkle with a pinch of salt. (Make sure chickpeas are dry).
3. Roast in the oven for about 25 to 30 minutes, or until chickpeas are crispy and broccoli is tender and browned,

being sure to stir the broccoli mixture half way through.
4. Meanwhile, add quinoa to a medium pot over high heat with 1 ½ cups of water or vegetable broth. Bring to a boil. Then reduce heat to low and cook covered until all the water is absorbed, about 12 minutes.
5. Remove from heat and let quinoa cool slightly.
6. In a large mixing bowl, whisk the remaining oil, maple syrup, salt and dill (if using) until smooth and consistent.
7. Fold the quinoa into the dressing in the large bowl. Add in about ⅓ of the roasted broccoli and chickpea mixture along with the chopped parsley and mix until well combined.
8. For serving, portion quinoa into 2 very large portions (or about 4 smaller portions) and topped each portion with remaining roasted chickpeas and broccoli. Garnish with sliced parsley. Enjoy!

ROASTED TOFU & VEGETABLES

A really simple recipe that bakes while you prepare other things. Enjoy this tofu and vegetables dish at lunch or dinner.

SERVINGS
4

PREP TIME
10 MINS

COOK TIME
40 MINS

1 package Extra-Firm Tofu
½ head Broccoli, cut into 1-inch florets
½ head Cauliflower, cut into 2-inch florets
3 large Carrots, cut into ¾-inch chunks
½ pound Brussels Sprouts, halved
3 Parsnips, cut in chunks
3 tablespoons Extra Virgin Olive Oil
Salt, to taste

Directions

1. Preheat oven to 400°F (205 degrees C). Drain the tofu and pat very dry with a paper towel to absorb as much moisture as possible. Cut tofu into 1-inch cubes. Drizzle 1 tablespoon olive oil on a baking sheet, carefully add in the tofu and gently toss together to coat the tofu.
2. Bake tofu for about 15 minutes. Remove the baking sheet from the oven, and flip each of the tofu bites so that they can cook evenly on the other side. Return to the oven for

15-20 more minutes. Remove baking sheet from the oven.
3. In another baking sheet, toss vegetables with about 2 tablespoons of olive oil so that they are all evenly coated.
4. Roast vegetables for about 30 minutes. Then take a look at the vegetables. (The parsnip and carrots may need a little more time). Remove any vegetables that are cooked through.
5. If the carrots and parsnips need more cooking, you can increase oven temperature to 450°F to finish them off. Roast for an additional 10-15 minutes.
6. Season with salt and serve.

CHICKPEA KALE & QUINOA STEW

This vegetarian stew provides nutrients from kale and proteins from chickpeas, which makes this dish a very nutritious and healthy one.

SERVINGS
2

PREP TIME
15 MINS

COOK TIME
35 MINS

5 ounces Fresh Kale, chopped
1 can Organic Chickpeas, drained and rinsed well
¾ cup Quinoa, rinsed and drained
3 small Carrots, peeled, sliced ½-inch thick
½ tablespoon Fresh Rosemary, finely chopped
½ small Leek, sliced and well rinsed
½ teaspoon Freshly Ground Cumin
3 cups Low-sodium Vegetable Broth (see page 228)
1 tablespoon Extra Virgin Olive Oil
Salt, to taste

Directions

1. In a food processor or blender, puree half the chickpeas with 1 cup vegetable broth.
2. Add the chickpea puree, remaining 2 cups vegetable broth, quinoa, carrots, leek, rosemary and cumin to a pot. Season with salt and bring to a boil. Add the kale and

reduce the heat to medium-low. Cover and simmer, stirring occasionally, until the kale wilts, about 12 minutes.
3. Stir in the remaining chickpeas. Cover and simmer until the chickpeas are heated through and the carrots are tender, about 5 minutes.
4. Season with salt and serve warm.

SAUTÉED POTATOES

A very simple sautéed potatoes side dish. Perfect to accompany poultry or seafood dishes.

SERVINGS 2

PREP TIME 10 MINS

COOK TIME 40 MINS

2 pounds Red or White Potatoes
2 tablespoons Extra Virgin Olive Oil
2 tablespoons Fresh Parsley, chopped
½ teaspoon Salt

Directions

1. Wash the potatoes thoroughly and place them in a saucepan. Cover with cold water and bring to a boil. Cook potatoes until they are tender, for about 25 to 30 minutes.
2. Drain potatoes and let to cool slightly. Once potatoes are cool enough to handle, peel them and cut them into 1 - ½-inch cubes.
3. In a large nonstick skillet, heat olive oil over medium heat.
4. Add the potatoes and cook, turning, until browned on both sides, about 10 minutes.
5. Add the parsley and salt and mix them in gently. Sauté the potatoes for about 10 to 15 seconds longer. Serve and enjoy.

RED LENTILS & VEGGIE STEW

This comforting lentil stew with vegetables is the perfect meal for dinner on a cold winter night.

SERVINGS 2

PREP TIME 15 MINS

COOK TIME 45 MINS

1 Bay Leaf
½ cup Red Lentils, rinsed
1 small Carrot, peeled and chopped
3 cups Low-sodium Vegetable Broth (see page 228)
2 teaspoons Extra Virgin Olive Oil
1 cup Fresh Spinach, torn
½ Celery Stalk, chopped
½ Sprig Fresh Oregano
½ Sprig Fresh Cilantro
Salt, to taste

Directions

1. In a medium saucepan, heat oil on medium-high heat. Add celery and carrot and cook for about 4 to 5 minutes.
2. Add lentils, broth, bay leaf and herbs and bring to a boil. Reduce the heat to low. Cover and simmer 30 to 35 minutes. Discard bay leaf and herbs.
3. Stir in spinach and simmer for further 10 minutes. Season with salt and serve warm.

TOFU WITH RED LENTILS

A tasty vegetarian dish loaded with lean protein from red lentils and tofu.

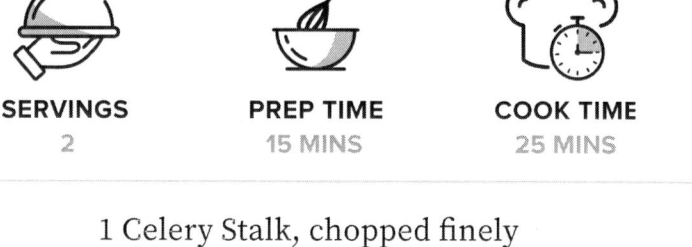

SERVINGS
2

PREP TIME
15 MINS

COOK TIME
25 MINS

1 Celery Stalk, chopped finely
½ cup Red Lentils, rinsed and drained
2 ½ cups Low-sodium Vegetable Broth (see page 228)
½ cup Extra-Firm Tofu, drained and cubed into ½-inch size
2 teaspoons Extra Virgin Olive Oil, divided
½ teaspoon Ground Cumin
Salt, to taste

Directions

1. In a saucepan, heat 1 teaspoon oil over medium heat. Add celery and sauté for about 4-5 minutes. Add broth and red lentils and bring to a boil. Reduce the heat to low and simmer for about 15-20 minutes.
2. In a skillet, heat remaining oil over medium heat. Add tofu and sauté for about 3-4 minutes. Sprinkle with salt and cook for further 1 to 2 minutes.
3. Transfer the tofu mixture into the saucepan with red lentils. Reduce heat to medium and cook for about 5 minutes. Serve while warm and enjoy.

WHITE & WILD RICE PILAF

This recipe features both white and wild rice, flavored with aromatic herbs to make a super-side dish to complement your main course.

SERVINGS: 8
PREP TIME: 20 MINS
COOK TIME: 45 MINS

1 Celery Stalk, sliced
1 large Carrot, chopped
½ cup Uncooked Wild Rice
1 cup Uncooked White rice
3 ½ cups Low-sodium Vegetable Broth (see page 228)
2 tablespoons Fresh Parsley, chopped
½ teaspoon Dried Rosemary, crushed
1 tablespoon Extra Virgin Olive Oil

Directions

1. Heat the oil in a nonstick, deep skillet over medium heat. Add the celery, carrot and rosemary and cook until the vegetables are tender.
2. Stir the broth and wild rice in the skillet and bring to a boil. Reduce the heat to low. Cover and cook for about 25 minutes.
3. Stir in the white rice. Cover and cook for 20 minutes or until the rice is tender. Sprinkle with the parsley and serve.

CARROT PATTIES

These wonderful carrot patties are very tasty, and they are also a healthy alternative to meat patties.

SERVINGS	PREP TIME	COOK TIME
2	10 MINS	6 MINS

1 Egg, beaten
1 cup Carrots, diced
½ cup Fresh Spinach, torn
3 tablespoons Non-Dairy Plain Yogurt
¾ cup Gluten Free Breadcrumbs
2 tablespoons Fresh Basil Leaves, diced
3 teaspoons Extra Virgin Olive Oil
½ teaspoon Cumin
Salt, to taste

Directions

1. In a nonstick skillet, heat 1 teaspoon of oil over medium heat. Add the spinach and sauté for 2 minutes until wilted.
2. In a food processor, add the carrots and pulse until chopped. Add the remaining ingredients (except the oil) and pulse until just combined. Transfer the mixture into a bowl and refrigerate for about 20-25 minutes.
3. Form the carrot mixture into your desired patty size.
4. In a large nonstick skillet, heat the remaining oil and cook the patties for 3 to 4 minutes per each side.

ROASTED CARROTS & FENNEL

A simple recipe of roasted carrots with fennel you can enjoy with the whole family. Roasted carrots give a colorful touch to this delicious dish.

SERVINGS
2

PREP TIME
10 MINS

COOK TIME
40 MINS

2 Bulbs Baby Fennel
1 Bunch Baby Carrots, peeled and trimmed
1 tablespoon Extra Virgin Olive Oil
½ cup Low-sodium Vegetable Broth (see page 228)
2 Sprigs Fresh Rosemary
2 tablespoons Quinoa
Salt, to taste

Directions

1. Preheat the oven to 390°F (200 degrees C). Lightly grease a roasting pan.
2. Cut fennel bulbs into 1-inch thick, lengthwise, keeping it intact from the root. Place carrots, fennels bulbs and rosemary sprigs in prepared roasting pan.
3. Sprinkle salt and quinoa over the vegetables. Pour olive oil and broth over vegetables.
4. Roast for about 40 minutes, tossing after 20 minutes. Serve while warm.

TOFU QUINOA STIR FRY

A healthy, vegetarian and gluten-free quinoa stir-fry made with crispy bake tofu, steamed broccoli and coconut sauce.

SERVINGS
2

PREP TIME
15 MINS

COOK TIME
35 MINS

1-1 ½ cups Cooked Quinoa
½ block Extra Firm Tofu
½ Carrot, cut into matchsticks
1 ½ cups Broccoli, cut into florets
2 teaspoons tablespoon Sesame Oil
2 tablespoons Coconut Aminos or Bragg's Liquid Aminos
1 tablespoon Fresh Parsley, chopped
¼ teaspoon Salt

Directions

1. Preheat oven to 400°F (205 degrees C). Cut the tofu into 1-inch cubes. Place on a baking sheet and bake for about 25 to 35 minutes, until tofu has crisped up. Stir it around a few times so as not to burn it.
2. Meanwhile, place the broccoli florets in a steamer basket and steam until just tender. Remove from heat.
3. In a small bowl, whisk together the coconut aminos, sesame oil, and salt. Set aside.

4. When tofu is done baking, preheat a wok or a medium skillet over medium-high heat. Add carrot, broccoli, quinoa and tofu and cook for about 2 to 3 minutes until warm. Add the coconut sauce and parsley, and toss to coat. Cook for further 1-2 minutes.
5. Remove from the heat and transfer to bowls. Enjoy!

TOFU VEGETABLE SCRAMBLE

This vegan, veggie-packed alternative to scrambled eggs makes a terrific lunch or breakfast. Tofu scramble can be enjoyed as a quick meal, or served with toast.

SERVINGS	PREP TIME	COOK TIME
2	15 MINS	15 MINS

4 ounces Mushrooms, sliced
7-ounces Tofu, firm or extra-firm, crumbled
½ cup Spinach, leaves finely shredded
½ large Carrot, diced (or 1 cup matchstick carrots)
1 tablespoon Coconut Aminos
1 tablespoon Fresh Parsley, chopped
½ teaspoon Ground Cumin
⅛ teaspoon Ground Turmeric
Salt, to taste

Directions

1. In a nonstick skillet, heat the oil over medium-high heat. Add the carrots and mushrooms and cook until have softened.
2. Add the tofu and sprinkle with salt, cumin, turmeric and parsley. Cook, stirring constantly, until the tofu is hot throughout and spices are fragrant.

3. Reduce the heat to medium. Add the spinach and stir. Cover and cook, stirring every minute or so, until the spinach softens, about 3 to 5 minutes.
4. Add the coconut aminos, salt if needed and stir thoroughly. Cook for further one minute or two until heated through.
5. Serve warm and enjoy!

MUSHROOMS & QUINOA PILAF

Quinoa simmered in vegetable stock with brown mushrooms and fresh herbs makes a delightful side dish for a holiday meal.

SERVINGS
4

PREP TIME
15 MINS

COOK TIME
20 MINS

2 small Carrots, peeled and diced
1 cup Quinoa, pre-rinsed or rinsed
1 ⅔ cups Low-sodium Vegetable Broth (see page 228)
4 ounces Shiitake Mushrooms, stemmed and thinly sliced
3 tablespoons Extra Virgin Olive Oil, divided
½ small Leek, thinly sliced and well rinsed
¾ teaspoon Dried Thyme
½ teaspoon Ground Oregano
¼ cup Fresh Parsley, chopped
¼ cup Pecans, chopped
Salt, to taste

Directions

1. In a medium saucepan, combine quinoa, leek and vegetable broth. Bring to a boil, then reduce heat to low, cover and simmer until quinoa is cooked, about 15 minutes.
2. Meanwhile, heat 2 tablespoons of olive oil in a large skillet over medium heat. Add the carrots and thyme, and

cook for about 5 to 7 minutes until the carrots are tender. Add remaining tablespoon of olive oil, along with oregano and mushrooms. Cook, stirring continuously, until mushrooms are cooked through. Season vegetables with salt.

3. Add cooked quinoa to vegetables and stir in chopped parsley and pecans. Taste and adjust seasoning if necessary. Serve warm.

RICE AND LENTIL PILAF

This simple recipe combines rice, lentil, and vegetable broth to make a tasty dish!

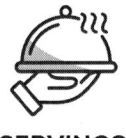

SERVINGS
2

PREP TIME
10 MINS

COOK TIME
30 MINS

¼ cup Lentils
¼ cup Uncooked White Rice
1 teaspoon Sesame Oil
1 Zucchini, cut into large dice
½ small Leek, thinly sliced and well rinsed
1 cup Low-sodium Vegetable Broth (see page 228)
½ teaspoon Dried Oregano
¼ teaspoon Salt
4 cups Water

Directions

1. Place 4 cups water in a medium stockpot over high heat and bring to a boil.
2. Add the lentils and cook until tender to bite, about 25 minutes.
3. Meanwhile, place the 1 cup vegetable broth in a small saucepan over high heat and bring to a boil. Add rice and leek. Reduce the until rice is at simmer and cook, covered,

for about 20 to 25 munutes until the water has evaporated. Remove from the heat.
4. In a medium nonstick skillet, place the sesame oil and add zucchini, oregano and salt. Cook, tossing frequently, until the zucchini begins to brown.
5. Drain the cooked lentils and add to the zucchini. Add the rice and stir until well combined. Serve and enjoy!

VEGGIE PATTIES

These vegetable patties are brimming with healthy ingredients that are flavorful and filling.

SERVINGS
4

PREP TIME
20 MINS

COOK TIME
30 MINS

2 large Eggs, beaten
¼ cup Almond or Coconut Flour
3 cups Fresh Baby Spinach, finely chopped
2 tablespoons Extra Virgin Olive Oil, divided
1 medium Parsnip, peeled and grated
½ cup Carrot, peeled and grated
½ teaspoon Ground Cumin
¼ small Leek, thinly sliced and well rinsed
¼ cup Kalamata Olive, finely diced
1 teaspoon Ground Oregano
½ teaspoon Salt

Directions

6. In a medium skillet, heat half of olive oil in over medium heat. Add the leek and cook until soft. Add spinach and stir until wilted. Remove from heat and transfer to a large bowl.
7. Add parsnip, carrot, oregano, cumin, and olives to the large bowl and mix to combine. Add the eggs and flour, and season with salt. Form the mixture into patties.
8. Heat remaining olive oil in a skillet over medium heat. When pan is hot (make sure it sizzles), place cakes in the pan and cook for 5 to 7 minutes on each side, or until browned and crispy. Serve warm and enjoy.

ROASTED SWEET POTATOES

This side dish is both deeply satisfying and nutritious. Sweet potatoes are rich in complex carbohydrates and fiber, giving them a low glycemic index.

SERVINGS 4
PREP TIME 15 MINS
COOK TIME 1 HOUR

1 ½ tablespoons Coconut Oil
1 ¾ pounds Sweet Potatoes, peeled, cut into ½-inch chunks
2 tablespoons Fresh Parsley, chopped
¼ teaspoon Fresh Nutmeg, grated (optional)
1 teaspoon Coconut Sugar
¾ teaspoon Salt

Directions

1. Heat oven to 350°F (175 degrees C).
2. In a small saucepan, melt the coconut oil over low heat.
3. In a large bowl, toss together sweet potatoes, coconut oil, sugar, salt and nutmeg (if using).
4. Spread the sweet potatoes in an even layer on a baking sheet. Roast, tossing occasionally, until soft and caramelized, about 1 hour.
5. Transfer to a large bowl. Toss with parsley and serve. Enjoy!

CRUNCHY CAULIFLOWER CASSEROLE

This loaded cauliflower casserole is unbelievably tasty, full of flavor, and tastes like loaded potatoes, but without all the carbs!

SERVINGS
4

PREP TIME
15 MINS

COOK TIME
45 MINS

¾ cup Slivered Almonds, sliced
1 head Cauliflower, cut into florets
1 tablespoon Extra Virgin Olive Oil
2 tablespoons Fresh Parsley, for garnish
½ cup Coconut Milk, full fat
½ teaspoon Ground Oregano
½ teaspoon Ground Cumin
¼ teaspoon Salt

Directions

1. Preheat oven to 400°F (205 degrees C). Put the cauliflower in a steamer basket and cook until tender. (It should be tender, but not mushy).
2. Put the cauliflower in a large mixing bowl and mash lightly. Add the olive oil, coconut milk and cumin and mix well. Season with salt and oregano.
3. Transfer mixture to a casserole dish and cover with foil. Bake for about 20 minutes. Remove from oven and sprinkle with the sliced almonds. Bake, uncovered, until almonds are toasted, about 10 minutes. Sprinkle with the chopped parsley if desired. Serve and enjoy!

ZUCCHINI AND POTATO BAKE

A very easy and delicious vegetarian dish that it's perfect to make as a side dish for summer barbecues.

SERVINGS
3

PREP TIME
15 MINS

COOK TIME
1 HOUR

2 medium Potatoes, peeled and cut into large chunks
1 medium Zucchini, quartered andcut into large pieces
¼ cup Gluten Free Breadcrumbs
2 tablespoons Extra Virgin Olive Oil
1 tablespoon Fresh Parsley, chopped
½ teaspoon Ground Oregano
Salt, to taste

Directions

1. Preheat oven to 400°F (200 degrees C).
2. In a medium baking sheet, toss together the potatoes, zucchini, breadcrumbs, parsley and olive oil. Season with salt and oregano.
3. Bake for about 1 hour, stirring occasionally, until potatoes are tender and lightly brown. Remove from the oven.
4. Serve and enjoy!

KALE AND COCONUT STIR FRY

A vegetarian stir fry made with sautéed kale, coconut flakes and rice. This dish is finished with coconut aminos and fresh cilantro.

SERVINGS: 2
PREP TIME: 15 MINS
COOK TIME: 10 MINS

2 cups Cooked White Rice
¾ cup Unsweetened Coconut Flakes
1 cup Carrots or Brussels Sprouts, thinly sliced
1 Bunch Kale, stems removed and leaves finely shredded
2 tablespoons Fresh Parsley, chopped
A handful of Fresh Cilantro, for garnish
2 Eggs, beaten with a dash of salt
3 tablespoons Coconut Oil
2 teaspoons Coconut Aminos
¼ teaspoon Salt

Directions

1. Heat 1 tablespoon coconut oil in a wok or nonstick skillet over medium-high heat. Pour in the eggs and cook, stirring occasionally, until the eggs are scrambled and lightly set. Transfer the eggs to a bowl. Wipe out the skillet if necessary with a paper towel.

2. Add 1 tablespoon oil to the skillet and add the parsley, kale and carrots. Cook until the vegetables are tender, stirring, for 30 seconds or longer. Season with salt. Continue to cook until the kale is wilted, stirring, about 2 minutes. Transfer the contents of the skillet to the bowl of eggs.
3. Add the remaining oil to the skillet. Pour in the coconut flakes and cook, stirring frequently, until the flakes are lightly golden. Add the rice to the skillet and cook, stirring occasionally, until the rice is hot, about 3 minutes.
4. Pour the contents of the bowl back into the skillet. Add the coconut aminos and stir to combine. Set aside.
5. Divide the stir-fry into individual bowls. Garnish with cilantro leaves.

SPINACH MASHED POTATOES

These mashed potatoes are such a classic and crowd favorite side dish. The spinach adds a great pop of color.

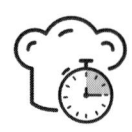

SERVINGS
4

PREP TIME
15 MINS

COOK TIME
25 MINS

1 pound Red or White Potatoes
1 tablespoon Extra Virgin Olive Oil
½ tablespoon Fresh Rosemary, minced
1 tablespoon Fresh Parsley, minced
1 (6-ounce) Bag Fresh Baby Spinach
¼ cup Coconut Milk
½ teaspoon Salt

Directions

1. Peel potatoes and cut into chunks. Place potatoes in a medium saucepan, cover with water and bring to a boil. Once water is boiling, reduce heat to maintain gentle simmer and cover saucepan. Cook potatoes until are tender, about 20 to 25 minutes.
2. Cook spinach until wilts, by either steaming or sautéing. Set aside.
3. Drain potatoes and mash them with a potato masher or fork in saucepan. Add milk, olive oil, rosemary, parsley and salt, and stir in gently.
4. Add spinach and mix it all together. Serve or keep warm in covered bowl set over pan of barely simmering water until ready to serve.

CHAPTER 10

SNACKS & SWEETS RECIPES

CAULIFLOWER SALMON BITES

These tasty cauliflower salmon bites incorporate eggs, fennel, and olive oil into a delicious snack. Serve with a little non-dairy yogurt and enjoy!

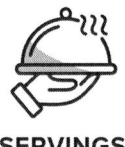

SERVINGS
24 BITES

PREP TIME
20 MINS

COOK TIME
20 MINS

2 Eggs, lightly beaten
½ cup Broiled Salmon, flaked
2 cups Roasted Cauliflower, pureed
¼ cup Fennel Bulb, finely chopped
¼ cup Leek, finely chopped
1 tablespoon Fennel Fronds, finely minced
1 tablespoon Extra Virgin Olive Oil
½ teaspoon Salt

Directions

5. Preheat oven to 350°F (175 degrees C). Brush a mini muffin pan with oil and set aside.
6. In a skillet, heat 1 tablespoon oil over medium heat. Add chopped fennel bulb and leek, season with salt and sauté for about 2 to 3 minutes. Set aside.
7. In a large mixing bowl, add cauliflower, salmon flakes, fennel and leek sauté, minced fennel fronds and eggs. Stir to combine. Then spoon rounded tablespoons of mixture into prepared muffin pan.
8. Bake for about 20 minutes or until golden. Cool and serve.

CARROT CAKE BALLS

These gluten-free carrot cake energy balls are quick to make, versatile, portable and you can pack them full of all the good things.

SERVINGS
14 BALLS

PREP TIME
10 MINS

COOK TIME
15 MINS

1 Egg White
¾ cup Pecans or Walnuts
2 tablespoons Ground Flaxseed
1 cup Baby Carrots
2 ⅔ tablespoons Coconut Flour
1 tablespoon Maple Syrup

Directions

1. Preheat oven to 350°F (175 degrees C). Line a baking sheet with parchment paper. Set aside.
2. Shred the baby carrots and pecans or walnuts in a food processor or blender. Place into a medium bowl.
3. Whisk egg white until frothy then add to bowl.
4. Add the coconut flour, ground flaxseed and maple syrup. Mix until well combined.
5. Scoop out 2-Tablespoon amounts using a cookie scooper, roll into balls with hands, and place directly onto the prepared baking sheet. Repeat until all mixture is used up.
6. Bake the balls for 12 to 15 minutes. Cool and serve.
7. Store refrigerated for up to a 5 days or freeze.

SWEET POTATO BISCUITS

Orange sweet potatoes give a soft texture and a beautiful golden color to these fluffy biscuits, which are perfect to serve with Thanksgiving dinner.

SERVINGS
9 BISCUITS

PREP TIME
10 MINS

COOK TIME
20 MINS

1 ½ cup Gluten Free Flour
¾ cup Cooked Sweet Potato, mashed
½ cup Unsweetened Almond Milk
1 tablespoon Baking Powder
1 tablespoon Coconut Sugar
4 tablespoons Coconut Oil
1 teaspoon Salt

Directions

1. Preheat oven to 425°F (220 degrees C) and place a rack in the center. Lightly grease a baking sheet with oil (preferably nonstick spray). Set aside.
2. In a medium bowl, mix together the sweet potato, coconut oil and ⅓ cup milk.
3. In a large bowl, add flour, baking powder, sugar, and salt. Stir just until combined. Add the sweet potato mixture and fold gently to combine. Slowly pour the remaining milk until all the flour is moistened.

4. Turn out dough onto a lightly floured surface. (The dough will be sticky so sprinkle flour on top of the dough too).
5. Knead the dough 10 times with palm of your hand until the mixture comes together, sprinkling with additional flour as necessary.
6. Roll the dough out to about 3/4-inch thick and cut with round or biscuit cutters.
7. Place on prepared baking sheet and bake for about 15-20 minutes or until golden brown and cooked through.
8. Serve these fluffy biscuits warm or at room temperature.

BAKED ZUCCHINI FRIES

A healthy and tasty alternative to the typical potato fries. These zucchini fries are crispy, flavorful and addictive.

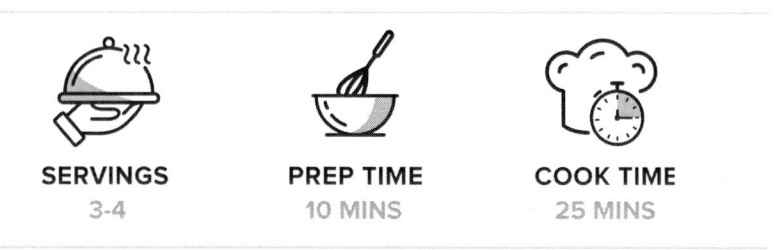

SERVINGS 3-4

PREP TIME 10 MINS

COOK TIME 25 MINS

2 medium Zucchini
2 large Eggs
¾ cup Gluten-free Panko Breadcrumbs
½ cup Dairy-free Parmesan Cheese or ¼ cup Nutritional Yeast
2 tablespoons Dried Oregano
½ teaspoon Salt

Directions

1. Preheat oven to 425°F (220 degrees C). Line and lightly grease a baking sheet. Set aside.
2. Cut each zucchini in half lengthtwise, then half again, then into quarters. You should have 16 slices per zucchini.
3. In a medium mixing bowl, combine panko, dairy-free parmesan, oregano, and salt. Whisk eggs in a separate bowl.
4. Dip zucchini sticks in eggs, coating evenly, and then toss in bread crumb mixture.
5. Place the zucchini fries on the prepared baking sheet in single layer without touching. Bake for about 20-25 minutes or until golden brown. Serve and enjoy!

AVOCADO WEDGES

Fresh sliced avocado, coated in crispy breadcrumbs and baked to perfection. These avocado wedges are incredibly tasty and easy to make.

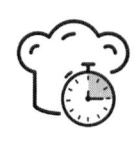

SERVINGS
2

PREP TIME
15 MINS

COOK TIME
12 MINS

1 Egg, lightly beaten
1 cup Gluten Free Breadcrumbs
1 Avocado, cut into wedges
⅓ cup Non-Dairy Plain Yogurt
½ tablespoon Cilantro, finely chopped
¼ teaspoon Ground Cumin
Salt, to taste

Directions

1. Preheat oven to 240 or 220°C fan-forced. Line a baking sheet with parchment paper.
2. Place breadcrumbs in a shallow plate. Place egg in a second shallow plate. Dip avocado in egg to coat, then dip in breadcrumbs to coat. Place on prepared baking sheet. Spray with cooking oil and season with salt. Bake for about 10-12 minutes or until golden and crisp.
3. Meanwhile, combine the yogurt, cilantro and cumin for dipping sauce. Season with salt.
4. Serve chips with dipping sauce. Enjoy!

PRETZEL STICKS

These crunchy and toasty brown homemade pretzel sticks are ideal for snacking or dipping.

SERVINGS: 4 DOZEN
PREP TIME: 30 MINS
COOK TIME: 55 MINS

½ cup Tapioca Flour
¾ cup Gluten Free Oat Flour
1 teaspoon Baking Powder
1 tablespoon Coconut Sugar
3 tablespoons Baking Soda
2 tablespoons Non-dairy Milk
1 tablespoon Maple Syrup
Coarse Salt for Sprinkling
⅔ cup Boiling Water
½ teaspoon Salt

Directions

1. In a large mixing bowl, combine the flours, coconut sugar, baking powder, and salt. Stir to combine.
2. Add the boiling water. Mix well until form a cohesive dough. It shouldn't be sticky, if it is add a little more tapioca flour.
3. Divide the dough into small several balls and roll out

into thin ropes. Cut into sticks or twist into mini pretzel shapes.
4. Fill a shallow pan with water. Add the baking soda and bring to a boil. Once boiling, add some of the pretzels. Avoid overcrowding them.
5. Boil for about 30 seconds. Use a slotted spoon to remove from the water and spread onto 2-3 baking sheets lined with parchment paper. Avoid overcrowding them.
6. Continue until all pretzels have been boiled.
7. Preheat oven to 400°F (205 degrees C). Whisk together milk and maple syrup. Brush a thin layer on all the pretzels. Top with coarse salt.
8. Place the baking sheets in the oven and reduce the temperature to 325°F. Bake for about 50-55 minutes.
9. Remove from the oven and let them cool for at least 15 mins before eating.

Note
- They are best fresh. Keep in an airtight container.

AVOCADO CAROB PUDDING

A thick and creamy pudding that's rich, wholesome, and chocolate-like.

SERVINGS: 3
PREP TIME: 10 MINS
COOK TIME: N/A

2 ripe Avocados
2 tablespoons Maple Syrup
⅓ cup Carob Powder
1 tablespoon Coconut Oil
½ teaspoon Vanilla Extract
¼ cup Shredded Coconut Toasted (optional, for garnish)
Pinch of Sea Salt

Directions

1. Cut avocados in half and remove seeds. Scoop the creamy flesh into a blender, food processor, or mixing bowl (if using an immersion blender).
2. Add the remaining ingredients (except the shredded coconut) and blend on high until smooth and creamy. (You may need to scrape down the sides).
3. Serve as is, or transfer to the refrigerator for at least an hour. To serve, top with toasted coconut (if using). Enjoy!

BAKED POTATO CHIPS

These healthy homemade baked potato chips are crispy, easy to make, and will certainly serve to satisfy your craving for something crunchy.

SERVINGS
3

PREP TIME
10 MINS

COOK TIME
20 MINS

2 Russet Potatoes or 3 Yukon Gold Potatoes
2 tablespoons Extra Virgin Olive Oil
Kosher Salt, to taste

Directions

1. Preheat oven to 450°F (230 degrees C). Grease 2 large baking sheets with nonstick cooking spray.
2. Peel and cut the potatoes into thin slices (⅛ inch thick) with a mandoline slicer or knife.
3. Place the potato slices in a bowl of ice water for about 10 minutes to remove some of the excess starch. Drain and pat the slices dry with paper towels.
4. In a large mixing bowl, toss the potato slices together with the olive oil and salt to coat evenly. Then spread the potato slices in a single layer on the prepared baking sheets.
5. Bake for about 15-20 minutes until crispy and the edges are golden brown. Watch them carefully to avoid burning.
6. Remove from oven and sprinkle with salt to serve.

BANANA OAT BARS

This is a delicious on-the-go soft baked bar without the harmful additives of most commercial bars.

SERVINGS	PREP TIME	COOK TIME
12 BARS	15 MINS	20 MINS

1 Egg, lightly beaten
1 cup overripe Banana, mashed
2 ½ cups Gluten Free Rolled Oats
1 ¼ cups Gluten Free Oat Flour
¼ cup Coconut Oil, melted
½ cup Maple Syrup
1 teaspoon Vanilla Extract
½ teaspoon Salt

Directions

1. Preheat oven to 350°F (175°C). Put the oven rack in the middle position. Grease a 9x13-inch baking dish with oil.
2. In a large mixing bowl, mix together the mashed banana, coconut oil, maple syrup, egg, and vanilla.
3. In a separate bowl, whisk together the oats, flour, and salt. Pour the oat mixture into the banana mixture and stir until well combined.
4. Scrape the batter into prepared baking dish and smooth the top so that it is an even thickness. Bake for about 18-20 minutes or until the edges just start to turn golden brown. Let cool on a rack for about 10 minutes. Cut into bars.
5. Cool and store in an airtight container.

BANANA "NICE" CREAM

A delicious, healthy and dairy-free ice cream recipe. Frozen bananas are the secret to this creamy ice cream everyone will love!

SERVINGS	PREP TIME	COOK TIME
2	10 MINS	N/A

3 ripe bananas, frozen and sliced
1 or 2 tablespoons Unsweetened Almond Milk
2 tablespoons Carob Powder (optional)

Directions

1. Remove bananas from the freezer and let them thaw for a couple minutes.
2. Place the banana slices, milk and carob (if using) in a food processor or a high-speed blender, and blend until smooth and creamy.
3. Serve immediately or freeze for at least one hour (if you want your ice cream to have a firmer consistency).

Note

- If you want you can also add 2 or 3 pitted dates and 1-2 teaspoons of peanut or almond.

HERBED CRACKERS

These homemade crunchy crackers flavored with rosemary are delicious and perfect for snacking.

SERVINGS
4

PREP TIME
10 MINS

COOK TIME
15 MINS

1 cup Gluten Free Flour Blend
1 teaspoon Fresh Rosemary, chopped
3 tablespoons Organic Shortening, cut into small pieces
½ teaspoon Baking Powder
⅓ cup Water
½ teaspoon Salt

Directions

1. Place an oven rack in the middle position. Preheat oven to 400 degrees F.
2. Combine dry ingredients in a mixing bowl or in a food processor. Whisk or pulse food processor to combine.
3. Add shortening. Cut in shortening until mixture is a coarse blend. Add water and stir or pulse food processor until a dough forms. (If the dough is too crumbly, add a bit more water.)
4. Roll dough into a ball and press between 2 pieces of parchment paper to ⅛-inch thickness. Remove top piece of

parchment paper and sprinkle with salt.

5. Transfer bottom piece with rolled out dough onto a baking sheet. Cut dough into 2-inch squares with a pizza cutter or knife.
6. Bake for about 12 to 20 minutes or until lightly golden. Let crackers cool before serving. Enjoy!

COCONUT ALMOND BUTTER BARS

These simple no-bake bars are perfect for an on-the-go breakfast or just as a lightly sweet snack to get you through the afternoon.

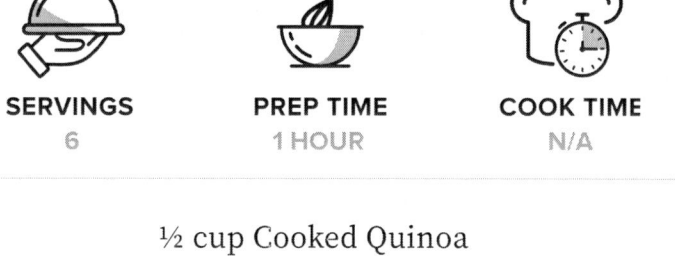

SERVINGS
6

PREP TIME
1 HOUR

COOK TIME
N/A

½ cup Cooked Quinoa
½ cup Almond Butter
2 tablespoons Coconut Oil, melted
¼ cup Unsweetened Shredded Coconut
1 teaspoon Vanilla Extract
1 ⅓ tablespoons Coconut Sugar
2 tablespoons Chia Seeds
¼ cup Unsweetened Coconut Flakes, toasted (see note)
¼ cup Coconut Milk

Directions

1. Grease a loaf pan with a bit of melted coconut oil. Then line pan with parchment paper and set aside.
2. In a small mixing bowl, add coconut milk, vanilla and coconut sugar, and whisk to combine. Set aside.
3. Place cooked quinoa, almond butter, shredded coconut and chia seeds in a food processor and process until well combined. Add coconut milk mixture and process until

combined. Then add the coconut oil and process again until just combined.
4. Press mixture into prepared loaf pan and sprinkle with toasted coconut flakes, pressing flakes gently into dough.
5. Place in freezer until set, about hour. Lift bar mixture out of loaf pan with parchment paper and slice into bars. Store bars in an airtight container in refrigerator or freezer. Enjoy!

Note

- To toast coconut flakes, place them on a baking sheet at 350°F (175 degrees C), for about 5-6 minutes.

BUCKWHEAT MUFFINS

These filling muffins are made with healthy, fiber rich buckwheat flour and sweetened with maple syrup.

SERVINGS
9 MUFFINS

PREP TIME
10 MINS

COOK TIME
15 MINS

1 Egg
1 small Red Apple, grated
¾ cup Buckwheat Flour
½ cup Almond Milk
3 tablespoons Coconut Oil
1 tablespoon Vanilla Extract
2 tablespoons Maple Syrup
1 tablespoon Baking Powder
3 tablespoons Unsweetened Coconut Flakes
¼ teaspoon Salt

Directions

1. Preheat oven to 350°F (175 degrees C). Grease about 9 muffin tin cups with oil. Set aside.
2. In a medium mixing bowl, add buckwheat flour, baking powder, and salt. Stir to combine.
3. In a separate bowl, add egg, almond milk, coconut oil, maple syrup and vanilla, and whisk until frothy.

4. Mix all the ingredients, along with the coconut flakes and grated red apple.
5. Divide the mixture into each cup of the prepared muffin tin. Bake for about 14-18 minutes or until muffins have browned around the edges and are firm to the touch.
6. Cool muffins in tin for about 10-15 minutes. Enjoy!

COCONUT CRACKERS & STICKS

These crispy coconut crackers and sticks make a wonderfully satisfying snack when paired with delicious mashed avocados.

SERVINGS
5

PREP TIME
20 MINS

COOK TIME
20 MINS

½ cup Coconut Flour
¼ cup Flaxseed Meal
½ cup Canned Coconut Milk (unsweetened)
¼ cup Coconut Oil, melted
½ teaspoon Salt

Directions

1. Preheat oven to 350°F (175 degrees C).
2. Into a medium bowl sift coconut flour. Add flaxseed meal and salt, and stir to combine.
3. In a small mixing bowl, add coconut milk and coconut oil, whisk to combine.
4. Pour wet ingredients into dry mixture, stir to combine.
5. Form dough into a ball and place onto a piece of parchment paper (approximately the size of your baking sheet). Flatten dough with your hands into a 7-8 inch square.
6. Cover dough with another piece of parchment paper

and with a rolling pin, roll to about a ¼ inch thickness. Cut dough into 2-inch squares with a pizza cutter or knife. Separate slightly and transfer parchment paper and crackers to a baking sheet. With remaining dough scraps, shape into pen shapes for sticks and place on baking sheet with crackers.
7. Bake for about 10 minutes. Remove any outer crackers and sticks that have browned nicely and sticks when ends are golden brown. Continue to bake remaining crackers and sticks for further 10 minutes, checking and removing crackers as edges begin to turn golden brown.
8. Remove from oven and allow crackers and sticks to cool before eating. Enjoy!

COCONUT CLOUDS

These coconut ginger cookies are light, delicious, and have a wonderful coconut flavor and are great for snacking.

SERVINGS 12
PREP TIME 10 MINS
COOK TIME 12 MINS

3 Egg Whites
1 cup Unsweetened Shredded Coconut
1 teaspoon Fresh Ginger, peeled and finely grated
1 tablespoon Vanilla Extract
1 cup Unsweetened Coconut Flakes
2 ½ tablespoons Coconut Sugar

Directions

1. Preheat oven to 350°F (177 degrees C). Line a baking sheet with parchment paper and set aside.
2. In a medium mixing bowl, whisk egg whites until light and foamy. Add ginger, sugar and vanilla, and whisk to combine. Fold in coconut flakes and shredded coconut until just combined.
3. Drop tablespoon size mounds of coconut mixture onto the prepared baking sheet. Bake for about 10-12 minutes or until cookies just begin to brown.
4. Cool on baking sheet for about 10 minutes before removing.

CHAPTER 11

ANTI-INFLAMMATORY SMOOTHIES

BANANA SPINACH SMOOTHIE

A healthy smoothie packed with banana and fresh spinach that provides your body several essential nutrients, and offers a number of health benefits.

SERVINGS: 1
PREP TIME: 5 MINS
COOK TIME: N/A

1 Frozen Banana
2 cups Fresh Spinach
1 ½ cup Unsweetened Almond Milk
1 teaspoon Fresh Ginger, peeled and grated
¼ teaspoon Ground Turmeric
1 teaspoon Ground Flaxseed

Directions

1. Place all ingredients in a blender and blend for several minutes until the mixture is smooth.
2. Pour into a glass and drink up. Enjoy!

PAPAYA MANGO SMOOTHIE

This smoothie is rich in antioxidant vitamins such as A, C and E. Papaya also contains the enzymes papain and chymopapain which help reduce inflammation.

SERVINGS
2

PREP TIME
10 MINS

COOK TIME
N/A

2 cups Papaya, chopped
¾ cup Fresh or Frozen Mango, minced
1 cup Unsweetened Almond Milk
1 teaspoon Ground Flaxseed or Flaxseed Oil
1 teaspoon Fresh Ginger, peeled and grated
¼ teaspoon Vanilla Extract (optional)

Directions

1. Place all ingredients in a blender and blend for 1 minute or until smooth.
2. Serve immediately or store in an airtight container for up to 1 day.

CARROT BANANA SMOOTHIE

A healthy, anti-inflammatory smoothie that will boost your energy and soothe your tummy. Carrots provide a lot of beta carotene to this smoothie.

SERVINGS	PREP TIME	COOK TIME
2	20 MINS	N/A

2 cups Carrots, chopped (about 275g)
1 ½ cups Filtered Water
1 large ripe Banana, sliced and frozen
1 cup Unsweetened Almond Milk
1 teaspoon Fresh Ginger, peeled and grated
¼ teaspoon Ground Turmeric

Directions

1. Make carrot juice by adding carrots and filtered water to a high-speed blender and blend on high until smooth. (Scrape down sides as needed and add more water if it has trouble blending).
2. Place a nut milk bag, strainer o filter over a mixing bowl and in the blended ingredients. Squeeze as much liquid out as possible. Transfer carrot juice to a mason jar (will keep for several days, though best when fresh).

3. Add the banana, milk, ½ cup carrot juice, ginger, turmeric and blend on high until smooth and creamy. Add more carrot juice or milk if it has trouble blending. Scrape down sides as needed.
4. Divide between two glasses and serve. Enjoy!

BERRY BEET SMOOTHIE

The color from this smoothie tells you that it's high in anthocyanins (flavonoid) that are believed to have strong antioxidant and anti-inflammatory properties.

SERVINGS	PREP TIME	COOK TIME
1	10 MINS	N/A

¼ cup Frozen Red Beet
1 cup Unsweetened Almond Milk
1 cup Frozen Berries (blueberries, strawberries, etc.)
2 teaspoons Maple Syrup
¼ teaspoon Ground Turmeric
1 teaspoon Fresh Ginger, peeled and grated
1 tablespoon Ground Chia Seeds

Directions

1. Place all ingredients in a blender and blend until smooth, adding more milk if needed.
2. Serve immediately, or store in a mason jar in the fridge for up to one day (for the best flavor).

PAPAYA GREEN SMOOTHIE

This smoothie combines spinach and papaya for a variety of nutrients, antioxidants, and digestive enzymes such as papain and chymopapain.

SERVINGS
1

PREP TIME
10 MINS

COOK TIME
N/A

½ cup Papaya, diced
1 cup Spinach, finely chopped
¼ cup Pear, peeled and cut into cubes
1 teaspoon Fresh Ginger, peeled and grated
6 Almonds soaked in hot water (to discard skin)
¼ teaspoon Ground Turmeric
½ cup Coconut Water
¼ cup Red Apple, diced

Directions

1. Place all ingredients in blender and blend for several minutes until smooth in consistency.
2. Pour into a glass and drink up. Enjoy!

BLUEBERRY SPINACH SMOOTHIE

A super green smoothie recipe made with spinach and blueberries for a powerful eye-opening anti-oxidant boost.

SERVINGS
1

PREP TIME
10 MINS

COOK TIME
N/A

½ medium Banana
½ cup Frozen Blueberries
½ cup Fresh Spinach, finely chopped
1 cup Unsweetened Coconut or Almond Milk
1 tablespoon Ground Flaxseed o Chia Seeds

Directions

1. Add all of the ingredients to a blender. and blend for 30 seconds, stir and blend for an additional 30 seconds.
2. Pour into a glass and serve immediately or refrigerate until ready to serve.

AVOCADO BERRY SMOOTHIE

This rich and creamy anti-inflammatory smoothie contains healthy fats and a lot of antioxidants from berries and kale.

SERVINGS
1

PREP TIME
5 MINS

COOK TIME
N/A

1 slice Avocado
1 cup Unsweetened Almond or Coconut Milk
1 handful Frozen Berries (blueberries, strawberries, etc.)
1 teaspoon Fresh Ginger, peeled and grated (optional)
1 tablespoon Ground Flaxseed
½ cup Kale leaves, chopped

Directions

1. Place all ingredients in a blender and blend for several minutes until smooth in consistency.
2. Pour into a glass and drink up. Enjoy!

APPLE GREEN SMOOTHIE

This refreshing apple green smoothie recipe is packed with a lot of nutrients and flavor.

SERVINGS	PREP TIME	COOK TIME
1	10 MINS	N/A

½ cup Spinach or Kale leaves, chopped
2 Red Apples, cored and cut into chunks
1 cup Unsweetened Almond Milk
¼ teaspoon Fresh Ginger, peeled and grated
1 tablespoon Ground Chia Seeds
½ Frozen Banana

Directions

1. Place all ingredients in a blender and blend for several minutes until smooth in consistency.
2. Serve immediately into a glass and drink up. Enjoy!

CARROT MANGO SMOOTHIE

The anti-inflammatory properties of ginger and turmeric make this a perfect anti-inflammatory smoothie recipe.

SERVINGS
1

PREP TIME
10 MINS

COOK TIME
N/A

1 large Mango, peeled and diced
1 small Carrot, peeled and quartered
1 Frozen Banana
½ cup Unsweetened Almond Milk
1 ¼ cups Water
1 teaspoon Fresh Ginger, peeled and grated
¼ teaspoon Ground Turmeric
1 tablespoon Maple Syrup

Directions:

1. Add carrot, banana, mango, ginger, almond milk, turmeric, maple syrup and water to a blender and pulse on high until completely pureed and smooth.
2. Serve immediately into a glass and drink up.

GINGER BERRY SMOOTHIE

Start your morning of right with this healthy smoothie which supports gut health and soothe your tummy.

SERVINGS
1

PREP TIME
5 MINS

COOK TIME
N/A

1 tablespoon Fresh Ginger, peeled and grated
1 cup Frozen Berries (blueberries, strawberries, etc.)
2 cups Fresh Spinach
1 Ripe Banana
½ cup Coconut Water or Alkaline Water

Directions

1. Place all ingredients in a blender and blend for 1 minute or until smooth.
2. Serve immediately or store in airtight container for up to 1 day.

CHAPTER 12

EXTRA RECIPES

HOMEMADE NON-DAIRY MILK

The possibilities of making homemade non-dairy milks are endless. They are easy to make, super healthy and taste incredible. You can make a variety of delicious and creamy plant-based "milks" by blending raw almonds, cashews, hazelnuts, sesame seeds, hemp seeds, flaxseeds, coconut, or oats.

SERVINGS
3-4 CUPS

PREP TIME
15 MINS

COOK TIME
N/A

1 cup Raw Nuts/Seeds/Gluten Free Rolled Oats or 2 cups Unsweetened Shredded Coconut
3 or 4 cups Filtered or Purified Water
Pinch of Sea Salt

Optional Add-ins:
2 tablespoons Maple Syrup or Coconut Sugar
1 teaspoon Vanilla Extract

Directions

1. Place nuts/seeds or oats in a medium bowl. Fill with 2-3 cups of water. Cover the bowl with a cloth and let sit overnight at room temperature. (Soaking time for cashews is only 2-3 hours. Hemp seeds, flax seeds, Brazil nuts, and shredded coconut do not require soaking. If using flaxseed, use only ⅓ cup).

2. Drain the soaked nuts/seeds/oats through a strainer and discard the soaking water. Then rinse them thoroughly under cool running water.
3. In a blender, add the nuts/seeds/oats or shredded coconut with add-ins (vanilla, salt, and maple syrup or coconut sugar) and 3 or 4 cups of filtered/purified water (depending on how thick you like your milk). Puree on high for 1-2 minutes.
4. Place an open nut milk bag (or 2 layers of cheesecloth) in a medium bowl, and pour the blended mixture into it carefully. Gather the nut milk bag or cheesecloth around the pulp and twist close. Then squeeze and press with clean hands until all of the liquid is extracted.
5. Transfer to an airtight glass jar or jug with lid, and store in the refrigerator for up to 4 days.

Notes

- It is advisable to use hot water with shredded coconut.
- Shake well before drinking, as it tends to separate.

HOMEMADE COCONUT YOGURT

This homemade coconut yogurt is a great choice for people avoiding commercial yogurt made from cow's milk. Enjoy with fruits or use in your savory recipes.

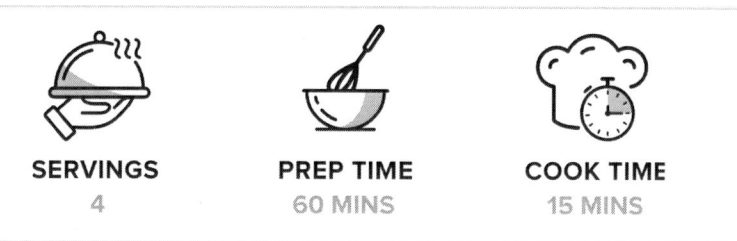

SERVINGS
4

PREP TIME
60 MINS

COOK TIME
15 MINS

2 cans (14 oz.) Full Fat Coconut Milk
1 ½ tablespoons Tapioca Starch
1 package Vegan Yogurt Starter or 4 tbsp. Non-Dairy Yogurt
1 tablespoon Maple Syrup or Coconut Sugar (Optional)

Directions

1. Sterilize your yogurt containers/jars, mixing spoons and other utensils by dousing in boiling water. (You can get mold if your equipment is not sterilized). Alternatively, you can run the containers/jars through the dishwasher.
2. In a medium saucepan, pour the coconut milk and maple syrup. Heat over medium heat until it reaches 150°F. (Using an instant-read thermometer is recommended).
3. In a small bowl, combine about ⅓ cup hot milk with the tapioca starch. Whisk together until the starch is dissolved. Then pour back into the saucepan of hot milk and whisk until smooth.
4. Continue to cook milk, stirring occasionally, for about

5-10 minutes, until the tapioca starch has thickened the mixture and registers between 180-185°F.

5. Transfer to a large glass bowl and allow milk to cool for about 30-60 minutes, or until the temperature reaches 110°F. (This step is very important as hot liquid will kill yogurt starter. Using a thermometer is strongly recommended).

6. Mix yogurt starter or 4 tablespoons non-dairy yogurt into a small amount of the cooled milk. Add to rest of the milk and whisk well. Pour the coconut milk mixture into sterilized glass jars with lids, and close the jars.

7. Incubate your yogurt at 110°F for about 8-14 hours. The longer you incubate it, the more tart it will become. **NOTE:** If you do not have a yogurt maker, here are some common ways to incubate your yogurt:

    - In the oven with an oven light on or proof setting (100°F). (I'm using this method for this recipe).
    - On a heating pad on low setting covered with towels.
    - In a crock cooker if you have a yogurt setting.
    - Using an Excalibur dehydrator set at about 105°F.

8. Place jars in the oven, close to the oven light (ideally with a 60-watt bulb). Turn the oven light on, and leave the yogurt in with the light on for about 8-14 hours. The temperature inside the oven should remain in the 100-110°F. temperature range. Use an oven thermometer to make sure. (Skip this step if you using a yogurt maker or another method to incubate your yogurt).

9. Transfer to the refrigerator and let cool for at least 8 hours. Yogurt will set as it cools.

10. Use in your savory dishes or enjoy as a dessert. Top with fresh fruits, a drizzle of maple syrup and some nuts. Always give the yogurt a good stir before eating. The yogurt will keep for up to five days in the refrigerator!

Notes

- If you don't have yogurt starter or non-dairy yogurt, you can also use probiotic capsules. For this recipe, use 3-4 probiotics capsules (opened).
- If you notice any foul odor, mold, or hints of pink or grey discoloration on its surface, that means bad bacteria colonized the batch, or that the starter culture died from temps too high or too low. Throw it out and try again!

HOMEMADE ALMOND MILK YOGURT

This homemade non-dairy yogurt is not only thick and creamy but it's also made with 100% homemade almond milk and packed with good bacteria that improve digestion.

SERVINGS 4
PREP TIME 60 MINS
COOK TIME 10 MINS

2 ½ cups Homemade Almond Milk (see page 218)
¼ teaspoon Xanthan Gum
1 teaspoon Locust Bean Gum
Pinch of Agar-Agar Powder
1 package Vegan Yogurt Starter or 2 tbsp. Non-Dairy Yogurt

Optional Add-ins:
2 teaspoons Maple Syrup
¼ teaspoon Vanilla Extract

Directions

1. Sterilize your yogurt containers/jars, mixing spoons and other utensils by dousing in boiling water. (You can get mold if your equipment is not sterilized). Alternatively, you can run the containers/jars through the dishwasher.
2. In a medium saucepan, combine the almond milk, xanthan gum, locust bean gum, and agar. If you want to make a

sweetened yogurt, also add the maple syrup and vanilla extract (omit sweeteners if you want a plain yogurt). Heat over medium heat until it reaches 185°F. Whisk constantly to make sure all the gums are dissolved and do not stay at the bottom. Remove from heat at soon as it reaches 185°F, just before it boils.

3. Transfer to a large glass bowl and allow milk to cool for about 30-60 minutes, or until the temperature reaches 110°F. (This step is very important as hot liquid will kill yogurt starter. Using a thermometer is strongly recommended).

4. Mix half a packet of the yogurt starter or 2 tablespoons non-dairy yogurt into a small amount of the cooled milk. Add to rest of the milk and whisk well. Pour the almond milk mixture into sterilized glass jars with lids, and close the jars.

5. Incubate your yogurt at 110°F for about 6–8 hours. The longer you incubate it, the more tart it will become. **NOTE:** If you do not have a yogurt maker, here are some common ways to incubate your yogurt:

    - In the oven with an oven light on or proof setting (100°F). (I'm using this method for this recipe).

    - On a heating pad on low setting covered with towels.

    - In a crock cooker if you have a yogurt setting.

    - Using an Excalibur dehydrator set at about 105°F.

6. Place jars in the oven, close to the oven light (ideally with a 60-watt bulb). Turn the oven light on, and leave the yogurt in with the light on for 6-8 hours. The temperature inside the oven should remain in the 100-110°F. temperature

range. Use an oven thermometer to make sure. (Skip this step if you using a yogurt maker or another method to incubate your yogurt).
7. Transfer to the refrigerator and let cool for at least 8 hours. Yogurt will set as it cools.
8. Use in your savory dishes or enjoy as a dessert. Top with fresh fruits, a drizzle of maple syrup and some nuts. Always give the yogurt a good stir before eating. The yogurt will keep for up to five days in the refrigerator!

Notes

- If you cannot find some thickeners mentioned above (such as locust bean gum and xanthan gum), you can omit them, and try adding ⅛ teaspoon agar-agar powder and ¾-1 tablespoon arrowroot starch to thick your yogurt. Do not add the arrowroot starch directly to the saucepan. First, mix arrowroot starch with ½ cup of milk. Whisk with a fork until incorporated. Then, pour the arrowroot mixture into the saucepan. Continue to whisk over medium heat for about 5 minutes.
- If you don't have yogurt starter or non-dairy yogurt, you can also use probiotic capsules. Use 3-4 probiotics capsules (opened) for both yogurt recipes.
- If you notice any foul odor, mold, or hints of pink or grey discoloration on its surface, that means bad bacteria colonized the batch, or that the starter culture died from temps too high or too low. Throw it out and try again!

HOMEMADE CHICKEN BROTH

A simple homemade broth rich in chicken flavor and lightly seasoned with herbs. You can use it in casseroles, soups, and other recipes that call for chicken broth.

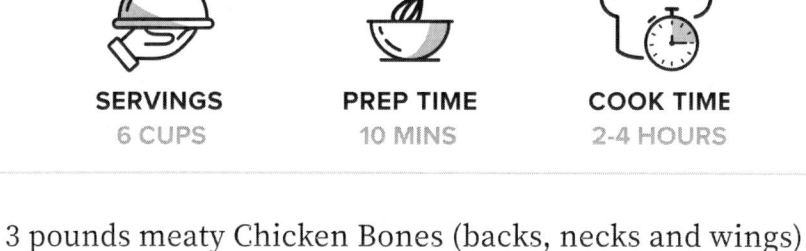

SERVINGS
6 CUPS

PREP TIME
10 MINS

COOK TIME
2-4 HOURS

3 pounds meaty Chicken Bones (backs, necks and wings)
5 Celery Stalks with leaves, cut into chunks
4 medium Carrots, peeled and cut into chunks
2 sprigs Fresh Thyme
2 sprigs Fresh Parsley
1 Bay Leaf
8 cups Water

Directions

1. Place all the ingredients in a large dutch oven or stock pot. Turn the heat to high and bring to a boil.
2. Turn the heat to a gentle simmer. Skim foam from the broth with a spoon or fine mesh strainer every so often when needed. Continue to simmer gently, uncovered, for about 2-4 hours.
3. Remove from heat and pour the broth through a fine-

meshed strainer into a large bowl or pot. Discard bones and vegetables.

4. Allow to cool for about half an hour, and then separate into storage containers. Refrigerate broth for up to a week or freeze it indefinitely. Remove fat from surface before using.

HOMEMADE VEGETABLE BROTH

This homemade broth will add flavor to your favorite vegetarian soups and stews. You can use this vegetable broth in any kind of recipe calling for broth.

SERVINGS	PREP TIME	COOK TIME
6 CUPS	10 MINS	1 HOUR

2 Celery Stalks, chopped

1 large Carrot, peeled and chopped

1 Leek, rinsed well and chopped (Optional)

3 sprigs Fresh Thyme

3 sprigs Fresh Parsley

2 Bay Leaves

8 cups Water

Directions

1. Place all the ingredients in a large dutch oven or stock pot. Turn the heat to high and bring to a boil.
2. Reduce heat to low and let your vegetable broth simmer for at least an hour, covered with a lid.
3. Remove from heat and pour the broth through a fine-meshed strainer into a large bowl or pot. Discard vegetables.
4. Allow to cool for about half an hour, and then separate into storage containers. Refrigerate broth for up to a week or freeze it indefinitely. Stir before using if broth separates.

THE ACTION PLAN

We have reached the final part of this book. Now all that is left is for you to take action. The first thing to do is to eliminate from your diet all the foods that can worsen your gastritis and trigger symptoms. In the fourth chapter (page 33), you found most of the foods you should avoid as well as those you should include in your diet. You also found general recommendations you should start following.

The consumption of foods rich in protein stimulates the production of stomach acid, which, along with the proteolytic enzyme pepsin, can irritate and damage the stomach lining. Therefore, it is recommended that you decrease your consumption of animal protein for a few weeks to reduce damage by stomach acid and pepsin.

As a substitute, you can take pea protein or hemp protein powder. These are two sources of plant-based proteins that are easy to digest. Hemp protein it is composed mainly of globular proteins (33% albumin and 66% edestin). Globular proteins dissolve easily so they are readily accessible for the body to use. Another option is to take a free-form amino acids supplement, which is easily absorbed and does not require stomach for digestion.

On the other hand, Sucralfate, which is a gastroprotective agent, protects the stomach lining by reacting with the stomach acid to form an adherent paste on the stomach lining. This prevents the back diffusion of hydrogen ions. It also absorbs pepsin and stimulates the production of gastroprotective agents such as prostaglandin E2 and gastric mucus. A natural alternative to sucralfate is DGL (deglycyrrhizinated licorice).

In addition, you can drink anti-inflammatory smoothies every day and introduce natural remedies such as aloe vera, nopal water, chamomile tea and supplements such as L-glutamine, DGL, slippery elm and probiotics to help heal the stomach lining. Zinc carnosine is another important supplement that you should seriously consider. It helps to enhance the integrity of the stomach lining and bolsters the ability to repair and protect itself. You may also find it helpful to take a powdered supplement containing L-glutamine, slippery elm, aloe vera powder and DGL at least two or three times a day (two hours after meals). Bone broth is very soothing and could be helpful, too.

Another extremely important factor is to reduce your stress and anxiety levels. Stress causes an excessive production of adrenaline and cortisol, which increases sympathetic activity. When stress is frequent, the body produces more than one hormone called cortisol; when the stressful situation persists for a long time, the body loses its capacity to produce cortisol and falls into extreme fatigue. Learn to relax using relaxation techniques such as deep breathing, meditation, yoga, etc.

The part of the nervous system that directs the body's resources to mental processes, repair, maintenance, digestion and rest is called the parasympathetic system, which is activated by a neurotransmitter called acetylcholine. A healthy nervous system balances its sympathetic and parasympathetic activities.

Regardless of the origin of your stress, when it is chronic, it can cause excessive activity in the sympathetic nervous system, an excessive production of cortisol and a deficiency in the parasympathetic nervous system's activity. All of this can result in dysfunctions, diseases, discomforts, attention deficit, fatigue and even memory loss.

For example, stomach acid is important for achieving good digestion, destroying the microbes and pathogens we ingest with food, and other functions. Its secretion results from the activity of the parasympathetic nervous system. However, if you are stressed all the time, parasympathetic activity decreases. This, in turn, decreases the secretion of stomach acid. The results may include gastritis, acid reflux, indigestion, IBS (irritable bowel syndrome), and autoimmune or inflammatory diseases.

If you feel stressed all the time, reduce your stress levels or avoid (as much as possible) any situation that can result in stress. This is as important as all the other things this book mentions; if you skip this step, you will be slowing down your stomach's recovery process.

Now that you know what you can do to start treating your gastritis, I want to share with you the following meal plan, which has been designed for those who prefer to follow a weekly meal plan without having to worry, every day, about what they are going to eat. However, it is not mandatory that you follow this meal plan. You can also customize it in your own way or use it as inspiration to create your own weekly meal plan.

One-Week Meal Plan

	MONDAY
Breakfast	Simple Oatmeal (see p. 56)
Morning Snack	Blueberry Almond Smoothie (see p. 62)
Lunch	Tilapia with Sautéed Kale (see p. 103)
Afternoon Snack	Baked Zucchini Fries (see p. 188)
Dinner	Creamy Broccoli Soup with Toast (see p. 142)

	TUESDAY
Breakfast	Spinach Mushroom Scrambled Eggs (see p. 58)
Morning Snack	1 slice Gluten-free Toast with ½ tbsp. Almond Butter
Lunch	Chicken & Veggie Stir-Fry (see p. 90)
Afternoon Snack	Papaya Mango Smoothie (see p. 207)
Dinner	Baked Fish with Carrots (see p. 95)

	WEDNESDAY
Breakfast	Simple Oatmeal (see p. 56)
Morning Snack	Banana Oat Bar (see p. 194)
Lunch	Almond Crusted Tilapia (see p. 120)
Afternoon Snack	Baked Potato Chips (see p. 193)
Dinner	Chicken & Veggie Stir-Fry (see p. 90)

THURSDAY

Breakfast	Pumpkin Spinach Smoothie (see p. 59)
Morning Snack	Papaya Mango Smoothie (see p. 207)
Lunch	Grilled Chicken with Spinach (see p. 106)
Afternoon Snack	1 slice Gluten-free Toast with ⅓ cup Mashed Avocado
Dinner	Roasted Winter Squash Soup (see p. 148)

FRIDAY

Breakfast	Spinach Mushroom Scrambled Eggs (see p. 58)
Morning Snack	Blueberry Almond Smoothie (see p. 62)
Lunch	Turkey with Kale (see p. 107)
Afternoon Snack	1 slice Gluten-free Toast with ½ tbsp. Almond Butter
Dinner	Grilled Chicken with Spinach (see p. 106)

SATURDAY

Breakfast	Blueberry Banana Smoothie Bowl (see p. 57)
Morning Snack	1 slice Gluten-free Toast with ⅓ cup Mashed Avocado
Lunch	Baked Salmon with Avocado (see p. 110)
Afternoon Snack	Banana "Nice" Cream (see p. 195)
Dinner	Tofu Quinoa Stir-Fry (see p. 168)

SUNDAY	
Breakfast	Banana Oat Pancakes (see p. 64)
Morning Snack	1-2 cups Fresh Fruits, chopped (papaya, cantaloupe, watermelon)
Lunch	Crispy Baked Cod (see p. 93)
Afternoon Snack	Avocado Carob Pudding (see p. 192)
Dinner	Coconut Chicken with Spinach (see p. 115)

Shopping List

Fruits

11 ripe banana
1 ripe bango
2 ½ pounds of papaya
½ pound of fresh fruits: cantaloupe or watermelon
3 ripe avocados

Vegetables and Herbs

3 medium Zucchini
1 pound broccoli florets
1 (10-ounce) bag spinach
1 small package mushroom
2 medium carrots
4 small carrots
2 russet or 3 yukon gold potatoes
1 small Butternut Squash
1 canned Pumpkin Purée
1 small bunch celery
1 small bunch leek
1 pound kale
1 small bunch fresh parsley
1 small bunch basil leaves
1 piece fresh ginger

Dried Herbs and Spices

1 small bottle dried rosemary
1 small bottle dried thyme
1 small bottle ground oregano
1 small bottle dried oregano
1 small bottle ground cumin

Poultry and Eggs

4 boneless, skinless chicken breast
½ pound lean ground turkey
10 eggs

Fish

2 cod fillets
4 tilapia fillets
2 salmon fillets

Seeds and Nuts

1 small bag chia seeds
1 small bag flaxseed meal
1 small bag pecans
1 small whole almonds

Breads and Grains

1 (10-ounce) bag gluten-free rolled oats
1 small bag gluten-free instant oats
1 small bag gluten-free oat flour
1 small quinoa package
1 loaf gluten-free bread
1 small bag gluten-free breadcrumbs

Dairy Alternatives

2 liters unsweetened almond milk
1 canned coconut milk

Condiments

1 bottle extra-virgin olive oil
1 (14-ounce) unrefined virgin coconut oil
1 can nonstick cooking spray
1 botttle coconut aminos or Bragg's liquid aminos
1 bottle toasted sesame oil
1 (4-ounce) bottle pure vanilla extract
1 (8-ounce) bottle pure maple syrup

Others

1 block extra firm tofu
1 small bag almond flour
1 small bag carob powder
1 (8-ounce) jar almond butter
1 (5-ounce) bottle dairy-free parmesan cheese, grated
1 container baking powder
1 small bag arrowroot flour or NON-GMO cornstarch

Tips for Meal Prep

Cooking more food at once makes it easier to put together healthy meals on hectic days. With a little planning, you can fit it into even the busiest week. The following actionable ideas will help you out to make the most of the time you spend in the kitchen. So, let's get started!

- Most of the included breakfast recipes are easy to prepare and won't take you long to prepare. However, if you desire, you can prepare some of these recipes the night before and store them in suitable containers (such as BPA-free plastic or glass food storage containers). Some of these are the recipe for Pumpkin Spinach Smoothie, Blueberry Banana Smoothie Bowl and Simple Oatmeal (oatmeal leftover can be store for the day you have to eat it again).

- You can take two or three days a week to prepare your lunches and dinners and store them in suitable containers for up to 3 days. Leftovers from Chicken & Veggie Stir-Fry and Grilled Chicken with Spinach recipes must be stored for eating on the appropriate day in the meal plan. Alternatively, you can prepare your meals the night before and store them in suitable containers so you can heat them up the next day or take them with you to work or wherever you go.

- Most snacks are also easy to make and won't take long to prepare, so you don't need to prepare them ahead of time. However, if you desire, you can prepare the smoothies and store them in a thermal bottle that you can take with you wherever you go. You can prepare the recipe for Banana Oat Bar in advance and store it in an airtight container. It is also recommended that you freeze bananas in advance to prepare Banana "Nice" Cream.

ABOUT THE AUTHOR

Paul Higgins is an avid health researcher and author of various books about different digestive disorders. He was diagnosed with bile reflux, acid reflux, chronic gastritis, and other digestive problems —such as dysbiosis and leaky gut— in early 2013.

During the course of about four years, he researched everything he could find about bile reflux, gastritis and the other digestive problems he was suffering. He learned how the digestive system works (including the physiology of gastrointestinal secretions), as well as how and why common digestive problems such as acid reflux, bile reflux and gastritis occur. He managed to heal his digestive problems through a therapeutic strategy with a holistic medical approach different from what conventional medicine offered him.

Now, this author of books helps other people who are also going through the same situation that he once went through. Through his books, Paul shares all the information, knowledge, and experience acquired over his four years of research on gastritis, acid and bile reflux, and other digestive problems.

Made in United States
North Haven, CT
02 November 2021